T0144843

BASIC HEALTH
PUBLICATIONS
USER'S GUIDE

TO
COMPLETE
SEXUAL
SATISFACTION

*Discover Natural Ways
to Encourage Intimacy
and Enhance Your
Sex Life.*

VICTORIA DOLBY TOEWS, M.P.H.

JACK CHALLEM Series Editor

The information contained in this book is based upon the research and personal and professional experiences of the author. It is not intended as a substitute for consulting with your physician or other healthcare provider. Any attempt to diagnose and treat an illness should be done under the direction of a healthcare professional.

The publisher does not advocate the use of any particular healthcare protocol but believes the information in this book should be available to the public. The publisher and author are not responsible for any adverse effects or consequences resulting from the use of the suggestions, preparations, or procedures discussed in this book. Should the reader have any questions concerning the appropriateness of any procedures or preparation mentioned, the author and the publisher strongly suggest consulting a professional healthcare advisor.

Series Editor: Jack Challem
Editor: Rowan Jacobson
Typesetter: Gary A. Rosenberg
Series Cover Designer: Mike Stromberg

Basic Health Publications User's Guides are published by Basic Health Publications, Inc.

CONTENTS

Introduction, 1

1. The Amorous Table, 4

2. Natural Aphrodisiacs, 12

3. The "Love Life" Lifestyle, 23

4. A Sexual Primer, 33

5. Creating Intimacy, 43

6. Erectile Dysfunction, 51

7. Infertility, 61

8. Talk to Your Doctor, 67

Conclusion, 79

Appendix: Common Medications with Sexual Side Effects, 81

Selected References, 83

Other Books and Resources, 86

Index, 88

INTRODUCTION

Sex captures our attention like almost nothing else, and for good reason—it's one of life's greatest pleasures. It is also an essential part of a fulfilling life—a great sex life helps us feel our best emotionally, mentally, and physically.

Along with thirst and hunger, sex is one of the most basic and powerful human urges, but sexual desire is much more than just a way to propagate the species. Sex is an expression of affection, a way to connect with a chosen partner, and a celebration of a joyful life. However, for all too many couples, the stress of daily life, the aging process, or declining health get in the way of a satisfying sex life. If you are one of the millions of people who find their sex life wanting, this book can help you reconnect with your sexual energy.

If you are reading this book, you may well be in a long-term committed relationship that doesn't quite have the pizzazz it once did. In the beginning, you and your lover probably needed nothing more than a glance from each other across a crowded room to start off a chain-reaction that ended in sexual fireworks. But as the years passed, children, careers, and the wears and tears of the body probably got in the way. Today you might feel like it takes nothing less than a nuclear reaction to get things moving in the bedroom. You may think this is the natural course of things, but it's not. Exciting sex does not have to be only a fond memory of your past; it can be a part of your present and future, too.

In this guide, you'll learn about the long and colorful history of foods used to fuel sexual fires in

Chapter 1. When it was introduced, Viagra became the best-selling new drug in history, and it continues to be a pharmaceutical superstar, even at ten dollars a pill. It's no wonder that natural (and cheaper) alternatives to Viagra—that is, herbs and supplements that serve as libido boosters—are a powerful part of the dietary supplement market. Chapter 2 will give a rundown of these natural aphrodisiacs and clearly explain which of these are worth a try.

But great sex takes more than popping a pill, which is why Chapter 3 details the lifestyle choices that sabotage your sexual energy and suggests activities you can do instead to keep at peak sexual functioning. For many people, however—nearly half of American women and a third of American men, in fact—the culprit isn't a lifestyle choice but a serious sexual health problem. These will be explained in Chapter 4, along with their treatments. And even when both partners are sexually healthy, poor relationship dynamics can scuttle any forays in the bedroom before they even get started. That is why Chapter 5 discusses creating the intimacy needed for good sex.

Chapters 6 and 7 delve more deeply into the physical problems associated with impotence and infertility. (Note that the old term "impotence" is being replaced by the more scientifically accurate "erectile dysfunction," or "ED" for short; those are the terms that will be used throughout this book.) In Chapter 8 you'll learn about the medical conditions that can interfere with libido, fertility, and ability to perform sexually. For instance, many people don't realize that medications are the culprit in as many as one in four cases of erectile dysfunction.

You'll see some specific warnings and contraindications with some of the herbs, supplements, and amino acids discussed in this book. In addition to these, please keep in mind that pregnant or breastfeeding women should not use any medication or medicinal supplement without their health care provider's input. And readers with specific health problems should work with their doctors to ensure that a particular supplement does not interfere with other conditions or treatments.

Finally, It is important to note that while sex is a wonderful experience, no one should put good health (or even life) on the line for it. Please practice safer sex by using a condom unless you are in a mutually monogamous relationship and know that neither of you has a sexually transmitted disease.

CHAPTER 1

THE AMOROUS TABLE

L ustful foods and potions have been a fascination of every culture throughout history, and with good reason—the line separating physical hunger and sexual hunger is often a very thin one. Many foods identified as aphrodisiacs fall into one of two categories: either they are reminiscent of the shape of genitalia, or they were rare or mysterious, which allowed all sorts of fantastic claims to be tied to them and not easily disproven.

Eating Your Way to Ecstasy

While some traditional aphrodisiacs seem to be simple folk superstitions, others have a clear underlying validity for the claims made about them. For instance, oysters are a rich source of zinc, a mineral that is necessary for optimal sperm and testosterone levels.

Testosterone
A hormone, best known for its masculinizing effects, made by both men and women that is an integral part of a hearty libido.

Eating in general can be erotic, as evidenced by the many shared meals that have served as preludes to other physical pleasures. Creating an intimate, sensual table from which to indulge is as important (if not more so) than the foods themselves. Candlelight should not be dismissed as a cliché; candles imbue a table with a magical, flickering atmosphere in which anything seems possible. As an added bonus, everyone looks better in candlelight.

Can you really eat your way to ecstasy with the help of chocolate or peaches? There is no hard evidence either way, but it can't hurt to try.

Alcohol

Alcoholic beverages are often consumed during a romantic meal to help set the mood. But alcohol has mixed results in the bedroom. While it lessens inhibitions, making men and women more receptive to sexual encounters, excessive amounts act as a depressant and interfere with the functioning of both male and female equipment. As Shakespeare's Macbeth so aptly comments, alcohol "provokes the desire, but it takes away the performance."

Alcohol in small to moderate amounts induces feelings of calmness and relaxation—essential precursors to being in the mood for sex. In addition, since alcohol dilates blood vessels, it may enhance erections and vaginal arousal. But there is a fine line between the prosexual effect of one or two drinks and the negative effects of more alcohol. Since alcohol is a central nervous system depressant, greater quantities can interfere with the ability of a man to maintain an erection and/or ejaculate. After three or four drinks, some men may not be able to achieve orgasm at all. Likewise, sexual response is compromised in women drinking these amounts.

Drinking alcohol can serve as the excuse people need to lower their inhibitions. If a person expects to have a sexual reaction to alcohol, he or she probably will. When a group of men was served a nonalcoholic drink, half the men were led to believe that the drink contained alcohol. The supposed alcohol-drinking group rated themselves higher in terms of sexual arousal and reported lower inhibitions toward sex. What this really shows is that the mind is the most powerful aphrodisiac of all.

A type of alcoholic beverage called mead has a long history as a fertility enhancer. Feasts, celebrations, and weddings in the Middle Ages all involved drinking mead. In fact, mead (wine made from honey) is the source of the term honeymoon: mead was used in a toast to send off the bride and groom after the wedding. The mead was believed to enhance virility and fertility. Many times the mead was credited if a baby arrived nine months later.

Beans

The reputation of beans was such that they were forbidden in nunneries under the rule of St. Jerome, who feared they would inflame the women's sexual senses. Lentils were thought by ancient Greeks to be particularly powerful in this way, while broad beans were the focus in Italy.

Chocolate

Eating chocolate releases the hormone phenylethylamine. The Aztec emperor Montezuma was purported to drink as many as fifty cups of chocolate every day in order to stay up to the job of servicing his harem. The great Italian lover Casanova was also a firm believer in the powers of chocolate. In the 1800s, chocolate was even prescribed by some doctors to patients seeking a boost in the bedroom. No wonder that Valentine's Day and chocolates are so firmly wedded.

Phenyl-ethylamine
A pleasure hormone released during sexual arousal; also found in chocolate.

In recent years it has become fashionable to claim that chocolate can be better and more satisfying than sex. If you know anyone making this claim, please give them a copy of this book! Chocolate is wonderful, and can be a fun complement to lovemaking, but those with a rich sex life know that no confection can match those feelings.

Fruit

Ever since Eve tempted Adam with an apple, fruits (especially those that are ripe and juicy) have had a sexual connotation. It only makes sense—fruits are, after all, the products of successful reproduction in the plant kingdom. Wonderful tastes and textures further seal the connection between fruit and physical pleasure, and, like chocolate, many fruits also contain the pleasure-inducing hormone phenyl-ethylamine. Think peaches, fresh figs, bananas, cherries, and mangoes.

Quince was dedicated by the ancient Greeks and Romans to their goddesses of love (Aphrodite and Venus, respectively). Some biblical scholars have suggested that the quince, and not the apple, was the forbidden fruit in the Garden of Eden. Traditionally, in Mediterranean wedding ceremonies quinces are used as a symbol of marital happiness.

Pomegranates were imbued with much erotic symbolism in the Middle East, where they were associated with fertility due to their abundance of bright red seeds. Pomegranate seeds were scattered during wedding festivities.

The eroticism of strawberries and other berries is closely linked to their appearance and to the provocative and messy way they are eaten by hand. Dipping them in chocolate can only increase their aphrodisiac powers.

Herbs and Spices

If your libido is in limbo, you might be able to spice up your love life with a few key herbs. A few hundred years ago in Europe, many spices were thought to have aphrodisiac qualities. In fact, children and young adults were cautioned to avoid spices (except salt and sugar) altogether. The spices most often singled out in this regard were cinnamon, nutmeg, ginger, cloves, mace, and pepper.

Of these, cinnamon is the oldest recorded aphrodisiac spice. Nutmeg and mace were combined in a drink for bridegrooms in the Middle Ages to enhance their wedding night performance. Saffron has been regarded as a supreme aphrodisiac, though most likely this is a result of its rarity. More recently, ginger was shown to improve the fertility of animals. Spices such as chilies and curries that raise the heart rate and induce sweating most likely were labeled love potions because the same physiological reactions occur during sex.

Festivals and celebrations of the ancient Egyptians and Greeks sometimes included fennel, which was linked to sexuality. For example, during the festivals associated with the Greek god Dionysus, fennel leaves were used as crowns and the leaves and seeds were consumed. The ancient Hindus concurred that fennel was amorous and prescribed an elixir for sexual vigor that included fennel juice.

The Romans consecrated garlic in honor of Ceres, the goddess of fertility. They also made a love-inspiring drink from pressed garlic juice and coriander. In the Middle Ages, garlic was purported to reverse erectile dysfunction induced by witchcraft.

Mint as an aphrodisiac was well-known in Shakespeare's time, and he wrote of it as a stimulant for middle-aged men. If nothing else, it does make for fresh, kissable breath.

See Chapter 2 for other, nonculinary herbs with aphrodisiac qualities.

Nuts

Pine nuts have been associated with sexuality for thousands of years, primarily in the Mediterranean region. For example, the Roman poet Ovid included pine nuts in his book *The Art of Love.* One explanation for pine nuts' love connection might be their high concentration of both zinc and arginine.

Arginine
An amino acid with a critical role in sex drive, sexual arousal, and sexual satisfaction in both men and women.

Walnuts have an erotic reputation, as well. Once again, the ancient Romans were the first to suggest that this food had romance-inspiring power. Walnuts were used in fertility rituals and also tossed at weddings the way rice is today.

Other nuts tied to increased ardor include almonds, pistachios, and sunflower seeds. There is even some animal research supporting the positive effects of some nuts, such as almonds, on sperm count and sperm motility.

Organs

The sex organs of certain powerful animals, such as tigers and bears, are believed by various cultures to augment sexual prowess. Other animal parts (such as rhinoceros horn) have also been thought of as aphrodisiacs. There is no evidence that these types of animal products impart any benefit whatsoever. In fact, many of these species, such as the rhinoceros and tiger, are now endangered, partially because they are in such demand as supposed sex tonics. Products from these creatures should never be used in any form.

Oysters

Oysters (along with truffles) are considered the most powerful of food aphrodisiacs. This connection goes all the way back to the myth that Aphrodite, the Greek goddess of love, sprang forth from the foaming sea on an oyster shell and then gave birth to Eros, the God of love. During the Roman Empire, oysters were so valued that they were purchased by their weight in gold. The famed lover Casanova was reputed to consume fifty raw oysters a day in his quest for sexual perfection. And he may not have been entirely misguided: Oysters do contain a great deal of zinc, a mineral crucial for sexual function. Deficiencies of zinc hinder fertility and hormone levels in both men and women. Just one oyster supplies most people's daily requirement for this mineral.

Truffles

The Romans were the first to promote truffles as aphrodisiacs, and since then this mushroom (along with oysters) has been credited as the ultimate aphrodisiac. After the Roman Empire fell, the aphrodisiac qualities of truffles were forgotten until the French revived erotic interest in them in the eighteenth century. The rarity and expense of truffles likely contributes to their ongoing connection to sexuality.

Vegetables

Artichokes have been considered an aphrodisiac over the years, but the provocative process of peeling off individual leaves and licking butter from your own (or someone else's!) sticky fingers is probably the primary culprit in its reputation.

Asparagus fits into the category of foods with a suggestive shape being linked to sexuality. Both the ancient Arabs and Greeks cultivated asparagus as a sex-promoting food. It was believed that a person who eats a lot of asparagus will also have a lot of lovers.

Celery has been said to increase arousal, and was at one time the most highly regarded aphrodisiac in Europe, where numerous folk songs allude to its erotic powers. During the Middle Ages, celery was used in charms to produce male children.

Eggplants, with their sensual color, sheen, and shape, were not surprisingly regarded traditionally as an aphrodisiac in medieval Europe.

Greeks, Romans, Egyptians, and Arabs all thought of onions as more than a spicy ingredient in their foods. At one time Egyptian priests were actually forbidden from eating onions, as it was thought that onions would interfere with their vows of celibacy. The Kama Sutra also includes numerous references to the powers of onions.

Kama Sutra The Hindu love manual, written in the second century A.D. in India, that detailed male and female anatomy, sexual positions, and techniques for enhancing sexual pleasure.

Potatoes were once strongly linked to sexuality, but this appears to have been due to their rarity. As they became a common food, their magic as an aphrodisiac quickly waned. Tomatoes, like the potato, also enjoyed a reputation as an aphrodisiac when they were first introduced to Europe. But there may have been more substance to this belief: tomatoes are abundant in lycopene, a micronutrient that may improve men's fertility.

The Bottom Line

While most of the food and beverages discussed in this chapter would be fun to include during a romantic meal, the following have the strongest erotic connections:

- Alcoholic beverages
- Chocolate
- Nuts
- Oysters
- Truffles

CHAPTER 2

NATURAL APHRODISIACS

The search for aphrodisiacs dates back millennia. Aphrodisiacs—named in honor of Aphrodite, the Greek goddess of love and beauty—work in many different ways. Some are tonics that crank up vitality; others more directly affect the reproductive system. And the most highly prized aphrodisiacs of all have a direct sparking effect on the libido, stirring desire and even improving performance and pleasure. Even though there may not be an actual "Love Potion #9," some libido-boosting nutrients and herbs appear to be the real deal. The vitamins, minerals, amino acids, and herbs described in this chapter have documented aphrodisiac abilities—just don't use them all at the same time. Be selective and choose the one or two that seem best suited to your situation. If those don't seem to work for you, move on and try a new one.

Arginine

The amino acid arginine has been tested for its ability to enhance arousal for both men and women. Arginine raises levels of nitric oxide in the blood and body tissues. This, in turn, increases the blood flow necessary for sexual arousal. In a study at New York University, fifteen men with erectile dysfunction were given dummy pills for two weeks, then a daily dose of 2,800 mg of arginine for two weeks. Six of the men reported improvement with

Nitric Oxide
A compound found in the body that activates other chemicals in the penis to initiate the muscular and blood vessel changes needed to get an erection.

the amino acid, but none reported any change while on the placebo.

Women also have something to gain from this amino acid. Arginine (given in combination with ginkgo, ginseng, damiana, and fourteen other vitamins and minerals) was compared to a placebo in ninety-three women lacking sexual desire. After four weeks, 62 percent of the arginine group reported significant improvement in their sexual satisfaction, compared to only 38 percent of the placebo group. Similarly, 64 percent of the arginine group reported a boost in sexual desire.

Arginine is found in protein-rich foods such as soy, brown rice, chicken, dairy products, and nuts. It is also available as a dietary supplement. A good recommendation is to take 2–5 grams of arginine in the evening or about an hour before a sexual encounter. If you suffer from bouts of cold sores or genital herpes you shouldn't take arginine supplements because they can stimulate the virus that causes those conditions.

Damiana

The reputation of the herb damiana as an erotic aid dates back to ancient times, particularly among the native peoples of Mexico. This herb is believed to be more appropriate for female libido problems.

In animal research, damiana extracts were found to increase mating behavior in "sexually sluggish" rats. In humans, the herb has been tested as a combination product along with arginine and several other herbs and nutrients. In one such placebo-controlled study of seventy-seven women with an interest in improving their sexual function, 74 percent reported improved satisfaction with their sex life, compared to 37 percent of the placebo group. Damiana can be taken about an hour before a sexual encounter.

Placebo
An inactive substance given to volunteers in a research study to compare results against an active substance given to other volunteers.

Supplement forms of damiana are generally taken in the amount of 400–800 mg three times per day. No significant side effects, aside from a mild laxative effect at very high doses, have been reported.

DHEA

The hormone testosterone has a powerful effect on the sex drive. The natural hormone DHEA serves as a precursor to testosterone, which is why this supplement is associated with boosting sex drive. The amount of DHEA in the body declines precipitously as we age, thus DHEA supplements can be especially effective for older men and women. One study involving older women (ages sixty to seventy-nine) found that 50 mg of DHEA taken daily over the course of a year significantly increased their libido. It is best to consult a doctor savvy in natural medicine before using DHEA; the doctor will most likely test your hormone levels to determine the best amount of this hormone for you to take (generally 5–15 mg for premenopausal women, up to 50 mg for postmenopausal women, and 10–50 mg for men). Amounts over 50 mg per day can cause acne, increased facial hair, and increased perspiration in some people.

Dong Quai

Dong quai (also called Chinese angelica) is often referred to as the "female ginseng." Traditionally, dong quai is believed to have a balancing, or *adaptogenic*, effect on the female hormonal system and to act as an all-purpose sexual and reproductive tonic. It has a long history of use in both Europe and Asia. In fact, it has been used in China for more than two thousand years as a tonic for women's reproductive systems, specifically for uterine bleeding, painful periods, and abnormal menstrual cycles. In modern

Adaptogens
Herbs that work as tonics to help the body adapt to all sorts of environmental stresses and to balance body processes.

times, herbalists continue to use dong quai for pre-menstrual syndrome, painful periods, and meno-pausal symptoms.

While dong quai is not a classic aphrodisiac, having no direct impact on libido, obviously having balanced hormones is a prerequisite to a healthy sex life, and this is where dong quai can have such a beneficial effect on female sexual desire. But men should not dismiss dong quai either. In a Korean study of Asian SS-cream (a nine-herb formula including dong quai and ginseng), the topical use of this cream was shown to delay orgasm over 80 percent of the time in men with premature ejaculation. Improvement was reported by 104 of the 106 participants.

Dong quai is not associated with side effects. As a supplement, it is generally used in the amount of 3–4 grams per day.

Ginkgo

The herb ginkgo is no Johnny-come-lately. This species is at least 200 million years old and individual trees can live for hundreds of years. As far back as 2,800 B.C., ginkgo was reported to have a medicinal effect in the Chinese Materia Medica (an herbal encyclopedia). In ancient times, the root and kernel of the fruit were used as a digestive aid, to support kidney function, and to nourish sexual vitality.

Only in the past few decades have the leaves of the ginkgo tree become the focus of natural medicine. An extract from these leaves has been widely studied for its ability to boost blood flow all over the body. In fact, ginkgo has become so well regarded in this ability that it is among the top few herbal medicines prescribed in Germany and France. Mostly, ginkgo is relied upon for its ability to increase blood flow in the brain. This improves memory and combats age-related cognitive disorders.

Just as ginkgo keeps the blood vessels flowing to the brain healthy, it also promotes healthy blood flow throughout the body, including the genitals in both men and women. As such, research has shown that ginkgo can be effective in some cases of erectile dysfunction. Researchers were intrigued by an anecdotal report of a person who had experienced antidepressant-induced low sex drive but recovered after taking ginkgo. A group of sixty-three men and women with the same problem were administered ginkgo (120 mg twice daily). The gingko showed positive results in 84 percent of the cases.

If you're interested in giving ginkgo a try, there are a few things you should keep in mind. Standardized herbal extracts are recommended in the amount of 120–240 mg per day. The safety profile of this herb is excellent, according to numerous large and well-conducted clinical trials. However, a few minor and rare side effects have been reported. Less than 1 percent of people enrolled in studies experienced mild stomach upset. Some people taking more than 240 mg per day of standardized extract have reported diarrhea, irritability, and restlessness. Mild headaches sometimes occur in those with poor blood flow to the brain, but only last the first few days of ginkgo use.

Standardized Herbal Extracts
Herbs processed to contain consistent levels of key active substances.

If aspirin is taken on an ongoing basis with ginkgo, there is an increased risk of bleeding, since both of these compounds thin the blood. Anyone taking a family of antidepressant medications called MAO inhibitors should avoid ginkgo, since ginkgo might increase amounts of MAO inhibitors in the brain to an unsafe level. Finally, those at risk for stroke or hemorrhage should not take ginkgo.

Ginseng

Ginseng is another long-respected herb, with a five-thousand-year-old reputation in China as a cure-all. In fact, ginseng root was so highly prized in ancient China that only emperors could collect the herb. Similarly, Ottoman Empire sultans boosted their sexual potency with ginseng. Current scientific evidence about the sexual powers of this herb suggests that the old stories might have something to them.

Ginseng is classified as an adaptogenic herb. This leads to the seemingly contradictory ability of ginseng to energize you when your energy flags, and relax you during times of anxiety. Ginseng also boosts production of sex-related hormones, such as testosterone, and aids in both male and female sexual response. Research has found that ginseng increases sperm production in men with low sperm counts.

There are three types of ginseng: Asian, Siberian, and American. The most commonly used ginseng is Asian ginseng, often labeled as Panax, Chinese, or Korean ginseng. American ginseng is closely related to Asian ginseng. Siberian ginseng, also called eleuthero, is not as closely related to the other two herbs, but generally has similar effects. Follow the label directions of each regarding how much to take as a supplement. Ginseng is a very safe herb to use. However, it can contribute to insomnia if taken too close to bedtime. Ginseng should not be taken by people with high blood pressure, diabetes (unless you work with your physician to adjust your insulin levels), or anyone taking MAO-inhibitor antidepressants or blood-thinning drugs.

Horny Goat Weed

Horny goat weed, also known as epimedium and yin yang huo, has a two-thousand-year history of use in traditional Chinese medicine. Legend has it that this aptly named herb gained its moniker when a goat herder noted the randy behavior of goats after they ate from a particular patch of weeds. It is reputed to be an aphrodisiac, although research on humans remains to be conducted. In theory, this herb works by increasing the levels of testosterone in the body. Further, horny goat weed may block an enzyme (acetylcholinesterase) that inactivates cholinergic neurotransmitters, which play a role in sexual arousal and performance. It is generally used in the amount of 1–3 grams taken about an hour before a sexual interlude; it can also be used on a daily basis as a general sex tonic. No significant side effects have been reported, but because it has not been carefully tested yet, it should be used with caution.

Kava

Since stress depletes the libido, improved stress management can help restore sexual desire. The anti-stress herb kava has been used for millennia by Pacific islanders, who macerate the root into a thick paste and drink it from coconut shells as part of a daily evening ritual. It produces physical and mental relaxation and feelings of well-being, all of which can promote an environment conducive to intimacy. Kava extracts can be taken in the amount of 200–250 mg of kavalactones (the active constituent) two to three times per day. Kava can cause mild stomach upset in a small number of people. Much higher amounts of kava are associated with more serious side effects and should not be taken.

Maca

Maca is a Peruvian plant that is eaten as a root vegetable or made into a fermented drink in the Andes. Maca's nutritional content is similar to corn, rice, and wheat, and superior to the potato for several minerals and protein. With such strong nutritional value, it comes as no surprise that maca is traditionally used to boost energy, stamina, endurance, and fertility. In rats, maca has been shown to improve sexual performance. In humans, this herb (1,500–3,000 mg per day) was documented to increase the quantity of semen, sperm count, and sperm motility. No significant side effects have been reported with its use.

Mucuna Pruriens

Mucuna pruriens (also known as velvet bean) is an herb indigenous to India. The Ayurvedic tradition

classifies this herb as an aphrodisiac. Mucuna pruriens has
been shown to increase testosterone levels, which may
boost libido. Additional research in humans is warranted,
but at this time there is not
enough information to make
recommendations.

Ayurveda
*A five-thousand-
year-old system of
healing developed in
India. It combines natural
therapies, such as herbs,
with a personalized
approach to the
treatment of
disease.*

Muira Puama

Muira puama, an herb derived from an Amazonian
bush, has some documentation as a sexual enhancer, which should come as no surprise since it goes
by the name "potency wood" in the Amazon. In
fact, muira puama is a staple of Amazonian folk
medicine, primarily as an aphrodisiac. In one study
with 202 women reporting low sex drive, a combination of muira puama and ginkgo resulted in
significant improvements in terms of desire, intercourse, and satisfaction with sex life. In another study
of 262 men experiencing erectile dysfunction and/
or a lack of desire, muira puama (in the amount of
1–1.5 grams daily) after only two weeks restored desire in 62 percent of the men and improved erectile
difficulties in 51 percent of the men.

No safety concerns have emerged with muira
puama. It is generally used as a standardized extract
in capsule form, 250 mg three times a day.

Oats

Oats have long been associated with virility, as cap-
tured vividly in the colloquialism
"sowing one's wild oats." Oats
were the focus of research in
the 1980s by the Institute for
Advanced Study of Human Sexuality in San Francisco, which
markets a line of oat products.
However, this research was not
published. At this time there is

Gluten
*A protein in oats,
wheat, and other
grains that causes an
allergic reaction in some
people, especially those
with a condition called
celiac disease.*

a lack of scientifically verifiable information about oats' effect on the libido. Nonetheless, many men and women take oat supplements and swear by the effects. Oats are exceedingly safe, unless you are allergic to oats or gluten.

Tribulus

The herb *Tribulus terrestris* has been valued in Ayurvedic medicine as an aphrodisiac. It is reputed to improve erections and prolong their duration. Protodioscin, a component derived from tribulus, was clinically shown to boost sexual desire and enhance erectile function. It can be tried in the amount of 1 gram per day. A few people experience stomach upset when using this herb.

Vitex

Vitex also goes by the name chaste tree berries, since it was at one time believed to quell sexual desire. Modern herbalists, however, believe that vitex does not result in chastity, but rather corrects hormone imbalances. In essence, vitex is thought to balance sexual energy, decreasing or increasing it as needed. Forty drops of the concentrated liquid herbal extract are combined with a glass of water and drunk in the morning. Vitex may take several months to show an effect, according to herbal experts. It should not be used by pregnant women.

Yohimbe

The yohimbe tree is native to West Africa, where it has been used for centuries to treat leprosy, coughs, and fevers. Westerners have known the sexual power of this tree bark for most of a century. Yohimbe is best known as an erection aid. Supplements are derived from the bark of the tree; a prescription medication made from the bark is called yohimbine (the name of the plant's active constituent). Yohimbe supplements work by dilating the blood vessels needed for an erection to occur. Research with men using 30 mg of yohimbine daily found this herb to be effective for erectile dysfunction.

Aside from the research focused on men with ED, there is traditional usage and clinical reports that yohimbe also increases libido and performance in healthy people. Although it has yet to be studied in women, this herb may well benefit women suffering from sexual dysfunction.

Despite the scientific and traditional evidence for yohimbe's efficacy, there are many cautions that should be heeded if you are interested in this herb. In fact, it is best used under the supervision of a health care provider. Limit yourself to 40 mg of yohimbine daily, since higher amounts can interfere with muscle function, cause chills or vertigo, or produce prolonged, painful erections. Some men taking too much yohimbe hallucinate or develop dizziness, nausea, insomnia, or anxiety. In addition, anyone taking yohimbe should avoid foods rich in tyramine, since this combination can theoretically cause dangerously high blood pressure.

Tyramine
An amino acid found in fermented or aged foods, such as cheese and red wine, as well as organ meats such as liver.

Dangerous Love: Aphrodisiacs to Avoid

Some love-potion peddlers stop at nothing to sell their sexual wares. Should you be wary of their wares? In some cases, yes. Certain reputed aphrodisiacs can be dangerous if used excessively, inappropriately, or even if they are used at all.

Spanish fly is probably the most famous aphrodisiac in Western history. Its use dates back to Roman times. It is made from an emerald-green beetle (not a fly) known as the blister beetle. The entire beetle is crushed and eaten, which causes an irritation to the urinary and genital tract. While this irritation can sometimes cause an erection, it is certainly no aphrodisiac! The end result is very uncomfortable and there are cases in which this legendary stuff has caused scarring of the urethra, infections, and even death. It should never be used.

In Southeast Asia, live beetles also are eaten as a folk remedy for lagging libido. Besides the fact that there is no evidence of this being effective, the beetles used for this purpose are a known host for human-infecting tapeworm.

A topical aphrodisiac made from toad venom has been associated with several severe illnesses and even death in men using products containing this substance.

An interesting report recently was published with a warning of sorts about the herb licorice. In men, eating exceptionally large quantities of licorice (seven grams daily) could increase a substance in the body that blocks testosterone production, thus contributing to sexual dysfunction.

The Bottom Line

For terrific sex, try these aphrodisiac supplements and herbs.

Men:	Women:
• Arginine	• Arginine
• Ginkgo	• Damiana
• Maca	• Ginkgo
• Muira puama	• Muira puama
• Tribulus	
• Yohimbe	

CHAPTER 3

THE "LOVE LIFE" LIFESTYLE

First the good news: Medical advances and the reduction of the stigma against discussing sexual problems have allowed sexual satisfaction to greatly increase over the past three decades. This increase in the number of sexually satisfied adults has been most pronounced among women, although women are still lagging a bit behind men in their level of contentment. And now for the bad news: There are still many sexual saboteurs out there, with stress, fatigue, smoking, obesity, and excessive alcohol topping the list. Read on to discover the lifestyle choices you can make to coax your mojo back.

Eat Right to Maximize Your Sex Life

To be able to fully love another person, you must first love yourself. Showing this self-love by caring for your body and keeping in good health is a great start. Nutritious food is the foundation for a healthy, sexy body.

One of the first things you'll want to consider about your diet is how much fat you eat, with the goal for most people being to reduce fat intake. There are so many ways that this one simple piece of advice will help your general health, as well as your sexual fitness. A high-fat diet contributes to high cholesterol, which clogs blood vessels, including those feeding the genitals. A high-fat diet also contributes to obesity, which in turn chips away at libido in numerous ways, such as lowering testosterone levels. Start small by skipping some fast-food visits and choosing foods in their whole form, as opposed to processed foods. Replace red meat with skinless chicken or fish. Use nonfat or reduced-fat dairy products.

The next big problem area for many people is not eating enough produce. If you're like most Americans, you don't come close to the recommended five daily servings of fruits and vegetables. Fruits and vegetables are low in fat and high in fiber—two qualities that help control weight and cholesterol levels and reduce your risk of cardiovascular disease. They are also treasure troves of vitamins, many of which are needed for a healthy reproductive system.

Another good dietary goal is to enjoy whole grains, nuts, and seeds. As with the fruits and vegetables, these are high in fiber and reduce the risk of heart disease. Choose brown rice over white rice, wholegrain bread in place of white bread, and so on. The key vitamins, minerals, and other nutrients in these healthy foods are an added bonus.

Move It or Lose It

No doubt about it: Exercising will make your sex life better. For men and women of all ages, those who are physically active enjoy more frequent and more satisfying sex. A good goal is thirty minutes of exercise, three or four times a week.

The improvement in cardiovascular fitness is one of the most important sexual benefits of exercise. This means that the genitals get the blood they need to function optimally. The cholesterol-lowering effect of exercise is another benefit, since cholesterol clogs arteries to the sex organs. Exercise even boosts production of key sex hormones. Exercise is also important because it builds endurance, flexibility, and muscle strength, all of which are valuable during active sex. Finally, exercise has many psychological benefits, such as boosting endorphins, relieving anxiety,

Endorphins
Brain chemicals that block pain, support a lusty sex drive, and bring on a state of euphoria.

and improving mood—making it all the more likely that you and your partner will want to make love in the first place.

How to Start an Exercise Routine

1. **Choose an activity that you enjoy** (walking, hiking, biking, skiing, swimming, and so on), and don't forget that sex itself is a form of exercise! For beginners, walking is often an ideal choice. You can do it inside (say, a mall) or outside, it doesn't require the purchase of special equipment, it doesn't take any special skills or abilities, it has a low risk of injuries, and you can do it alone or with a buddy.

2. **Don't push too hard at first.** Start slowly so that your body gets used to exercise and you aren't too sore to continue.

3. **Keep convenience in mind.** If you want to join a gym, choose one close to your home or office. Make sure you have exercise options that don't depend on a certain type of weather. You don't want any easy excuses to skip your exercise that day.

4. **Spice up your routine.** Don't sabotage yourself by only doing one class at the gym or only using one exercise machine at home. Rotate through different activities so that boredom doesn't stop you from exercising.

5. **Work out with a buddy.** This will help keep you motivated and lessen the chance that you'll skip the workout.

Bike Riding Caution

Riding a bicycle is great exercise, but there are a few cautions to keep in mind so that this form of exercise doesn't backfire and leave you with sexual problems. An accident (even as minor as a hard strike into a curb or a bump in the road) could cause you to slide forward on your seat and collide with the slender metal tube that runs between the seat and handlebar posts. This type of acute injury has been noted as being a potential cause of sexual difficulties, sometimes even when the injury occurred earlier in life.

A more disconcerting problem is a type of long-term damage caused by hard, narrow bicycle seats. These seats compress the arteries and nerves that lead to the genitals, cutting off blood flow and causing permanent tissue damage. This is primarily problematic for men: Half of hardcore male cyclists experience genital numbness, and twice as many cyclists have erectile dysfunction compared to men involved in different forms of exercise. In the United States, the number of cyclists suffering from, or at risk of, sexual dysfunction from this cause has been estimated to be as high as four million. The more miles in the saddle, the greater the chance of sexual injuries.

This does not mean that you have to give up bike riding; the health benefits of riding do outweigh the risks. Common sense also plays a role here. If you are experiencing any genital numbness or erectile dysfunction, stop riding. Otherwise, feel free to use bicycling as exercise. Recent improvements in bicycle seat design have also minimized the risks. New, U-shaped seats move the pressure off the penile artery. It's better to take multiple short rides, rather than fewer, long rides.

Consider Kegels

Engaging in exercise of any kind generally contributes to a better sex life, but a special type of exercise called Kegels can specifically improve sexual performance. Kegels focus on improving the muscle tone of a set of muscles in the genital region that rarely get attention otherwise. Kegel exercises were developed by a surgeon named Arnold Kegel in the 1950s with the goal

Pubococcygeal Muscles

Muscles located between the genitals and anus, used in reproduction and elimination functions.

to restore or improve the tone of the pubococ-cygeal muscles, otherwise known as the pelvic floor. The pelvic floor often weakens during pregnancy and childbirth, as well as during the older years as a result of the aging process.

To perform Kegel exercises, you squeeze together the muscles of the pelvic floor, as if you were trying to stop urine in midstream. Squeeze and release in sets of ten several times a day. This should strengthen muscle tone. Kegels are recommended for some women to prevent incontinence, but another benefit is improved sexual pleasure in many women. Doing Kegels during intercourse might also enhance pleasure for you and your partner.

The Perils of Stress

Stress is the nemesis of a healthy sex drive. The fight-or-flight response of adrenaline cuts blood flow to "nonessential" body parts, and in this case that includes the genitals. Being wound up about a challenging job situation, snarled traffic jams, or other hassles in life is not compatible with great sex. Since stress depletes the libido, practicing stress management techniques can have the side effect of restoring sexual ardor.

Managing Your Stress

Stress management techniques that calm the inner environment can go a long way in helping to deal with the hectic outside world. Meditation is one such coping mechanism that has both a long history of use and modern confirmation of effectiveness. By working to quiet the mind and body, meditation reduces the sometimes overwhelming stimulation that drives feelings of anxiety and stress. An easy approach to meditation is to sit or lie down in a dark room and then focus on a word or phrase as you breathe in and out deeply and evenly for about twenty minutes. You may find that afterward you have a whole new perspective on the things stressing you out.

Visualizing success is a great way to keep life light-hearted. Worrying—that is, letting your mind focus on what could go wrong in your life, instead of focusing on what might go right—unconsciously sets you up for failure and cranks up your anxiety level. Your body reacts to the mental imagery of losing your job, a conflict with your mate, or any other imagined problem as if the situation is actually happening; stress hormones are pumped out of your adrenals, your heart rate increases, and muscles tense. By directing your mental imagery toward visualizing success, your body relaxes, you feel better, and your unconscious mind works to reach these positive goals.

Adrenals
Glands above the kidneys that secrete hormones during times of stress to alter certain functions in the body, including raising heart rate and respiration.

And don't forget about one other stress reliever: sex. Sex is actually a very effective way to lower your stress level; you just have to find the time to partake in this pleasure.

Stress-Relieving Supplements

The anti-stress herb kava produces physical and mental relaxation and feelings of well-being, all of which promote an environment conducive to intimacy. Kava has only recently gained recognition for easing stress, tension, and anxiety in the Western world, but its traditional use as a social beverage in the Polynesian islands can be traced back three thousand years. Modern research reveals that kava root contains several active ingredients (known as kavalactones) that produce physical and mental relaxation and feelings of well-being. In fact, kava root extract is currently a commonly prescribed remedy for anxiety throughout Europe.

A thorough review of published kava research gave a thumbs-up for kava as an anti-anxiety tool. Repeatedly, kava was shown to be superior to dummy pills for the relief of anxiety. The majority of anxiety research is based on 100 mg capsules of kava (standardized to provide 70 mg of kavalactones), taken three times per day.

Side effects can occur with much higher doses of kava, but they are minor and include mild stomach upset and skin rashes. More serious skin problems do occur, however, in individuals using kava excessively over a long period of time; this should be avoided. Kava should not be used by pregnant or nursing women, or anyone taking antidepressants or other drugs that affect the central nervous system.

Stress and anxiety take their toll on mineral stores in the body. Type A people—highly energetic and aggressive individuals—have been found to have higher levels of stress hormones in their blood, yet lower levels of magnesium when compared to their more laid-back counterparts. As if that weren't enough, these stress hormones cause body cells to lose magnesium. And as the body's stores of magnesium are drained, the stress response is activated—leading to a stress spiral. All of this, of course, does not promote a sense of relaxation.

Most people do not reach recommended intake levels of magnesium in their diets. Foods rich in magnesium include green leafy vegetables, grains, and legumes. In terms of supplementation, 250–350 mg per day is probably a good range for most individuals.

The B-complex vitamins play a role in how well—or poorly—your body responds to the pressures of modern living. For starters, most of the B vitamins are involved in the development or maintenance of a well-functioning nervous system. B vitamins are also needed to manufacture certain neurotransmitters. B vitamins help ensure that the nervous system is up to the challenge of life's ups and downs. Since nutritional surveys suggest that many American diets fall short with several of the B vitamins, a balanced B-complex supplement

Neurotransmitters *Hormonelike chemicals used to convey messages between nerve cells.*

can be both a form of general nutritional insurance and a way to boost the body's resistance to the effects of stress.

Of the B-complex vitamins, vitamin B_3 in the form called niacinamide may be particularly beneficial, since it seems to affect the brain much like certain conventional anti-anxiety drugs, such as Valium. Supplements providing 500 mg of niacinamide, taken several times daily, can be used to ease anxiety and stress.

Smoking and Erectile Dysfunction

The verdict is in: Smoking is a health disaster. In addition to the well-known risks of lung cancer, emphysema, heart attack, and stroke, smoking can ruin your fun in the bedroom, too. Men who smoke cigarettes are *seven* times as likely to develop erectile dysfunction as nonsmoking men. It's ironic that classic movies often depict smoking as the natural follow-up to lovemaking when the reality is that, if you smoke, you are less likely even to be able to make love.

Smoking leads to ED as a result of restricted circulation. Although not yet well researched, female sexual response is probably also compromised, since pleasure in women also depends on good blood flow to the genitals. Only 28 percent of the general population smokes, but a whopping 40 percent of men with ED are smokers. Clearly, smoking wreaks havoc on the workings of male equipment. But even here there is some good news to share. Former smokers have no higher risk of erectile dysfunction than men who have never smoked. It's never too late to quit: for the sake of your sex life, heart, lungs, and life itself.

"Not Tonight, Dear, I'm Tired"

How often has fatigue prevented you or your partner from engaging in a bedtime romp? Fatigue is the killer of many couple's sex lives. Schedules are often so packed with work and family obligations that sex is simply crowded out of the day (or week, or even month).

Although eight hours of shut-eye is the standard recommendation, almost half of Americans sleep only six hours or less each night. Sleep deprivation saps your interest in many activities, including sex. Furthermore, lack of sleep is linked to depressed mood and crankiness, two qualities that don't endear themselves to high sexual interest, pleasure, and performance.

For one out of every three Americans, the problem is not finding the time to sleep, but actually falling or staying asleep. Insomnia is experienced by 95 percent of adults at some point in their lives. Insomnia varies in its severity. Transient insomnia lasts only a few nights and is often the result of excitement, minor stress, or caffeine intake. Short-term insomnia persists for a couple of weeks and stems from major stress or illness. Chronic insomnia is a long-term disorder with many contributing factors, including physical illness, depression, poor sleeping environment, and lifestyle. But any degree of insomnia can impact health and contribute to daytime drowsiness, irritability, low stress threshold—and no sex life.

About half of the cases of insomnia are caused by psychological and emotional stress. Feeling "wound up," juggling work and home life, or facing constant deadlines makes for restless bedfellows. To complicate matters, stress in itself contributes to insomnia, so a viscous cycle of worsening sleep deprivation can develop. Relaxation should be the first ingredient in a successful formula for a good night's sleep. See the earlier recommendations in this book for exercise and stress-management.

Weight Management

Your weight plays a role in sexual health. Carrying around a few extra pounds is not an issue, but being either severely overweight or underweight both have negative consequences. High blood pressure and high cholesterol associated with obesity can in turn lead to sexual dysfunction, while being significantly underweight can jeopardize sexual function and fertility through anemia, fatigue, and impaired hormone production.

When getting in shape, there is no need to strive for the unrealistic Hollywood hardbody. In fact, a man or a woman who is content with his or her body, despite a few extra pounds, is much more attractive than a person who is obsessed with weight. Nevertheless, being overweight can lead to negative body image and self-esteem. In such cases, losing weight can give a real boost to sexual passion and performance.

The Bottom Line

To keep your libido in tip-top shape you'll want to avoid sexual saboteurs.

- Fuel your body with good foods and you'll be better able to fuel your passions. Avoid excessive fat and instead pile on the produce.

- Partake in physical activity on a regular basis if you want to be able to "get physical."

- Stress saps sexual vigor; manage your stress with meditation, exercise, or supplements such as kava.

- Smoking is a surefire way to put out the bedroom fires; if you smoke, quit.

- Keep well-rested so that you have enough energy to play in bed and not just crash for the night.

- Obesity ups the chances for other health problems that interfere with sexual health. Keep yourself at a healthy weight.

CHAPTER 4

A SEXUAL PRIMER

To be a competent lover it is important to understand the basics about male and female sexual equipment and how the body reacts during a sexual encounter. This chapter covers that information, then goes on to explain the details of the many things that can go wrong with those systems.

Anatomy Basics

The male's sexual equipment consists of the penis, scrotum, and testicles. The penis, when not erect, is between two and four inches long in most men. It lengthens when erect to an average of six inches. This happens through basic hydraulics: the penis consists of three cylinders of spongy tissue packed together, two large cylinders on top and a smaller one underneath. The smaller cylinder carries the tubing for urine and semen. These cylinders become engorged with blood when a man is sexually aroused, which causes them to inflate and harden, just like a water balloon as it fills. The tip of the penis is called the glans and is highly sensitive. The scrotum is the skin-covered pouch that contains the testicles. The testicles produce sperm and secrete male hormones.

The female reproductive system consists of the external genitals (vulva) and internal genitals. The external genitals include the mons pubis, the outer fold of skin called the labia majora, the inner fold of skin called the labia minora, and the clitoris. The internal

Mons Pubis
The mound of nerve and fatty tissue that is covered by the woman's pubic hair; it protects the pubic bone.

genitals include the vagina, uterus, fallopian tubes, and ovaries.

How Arousal Happens

Sexual arousal is a complex process involving the brain, nervous system, hormones, and genitals. The sexual response cycle is essentially the same for men and women and consists of four stages: desire, arousal, orgasm, and resolution.

In the desire stage, both men and women experience a rush of blood that engorges the genitals. In men, this is evidenced by an erection, when the arteries of the penis relax and widen to allow in extra blood. Meanwhile, the veins that normally carry blood away from the penis are compressed to trap the blood in the penis. The testicles are drawn closer to the body. A woman's clitoris becomes erect, her labia swell, the vaginal walls expand, and vaginal lubrication begins. Both genders experience an increase in muscle tension, hardening nipples, and increased heart rate.

Clitoris
The highly sensitive organ located just below the mons pubis at the top of the labia minora. Its sole purpose is to provide sexual stimulation and pleasure.

The arousal stage is in essence a continuation of the desire stage, during which there is an increase in feelings of sexual tension. The penis continues to increase in size, the testicles move even higher, and a small amount of fluid might be expelled from the penis. For women, the vagina continues to expand, the clitoris retracts, and the breasts become larger. Both men and women might develop sex flush—a darkening of the skin on the upper chest, neck, and face, rapid breathing, fast pulse, and rise in blood pressure.

The orgasm stage needs no explanation for most people; it is the extremely pleasurable contractions that culminate a sexual experience and release the muscle tension that had been building. At this point, a man ejaculates.

In the resolution stage, the congestion of blood at various parts of the body dissipates and muscles that were previously tensed become relaxed again. The penis becomes flaccid, heart rate drops back to normal, and both partners essentially return to an unstimulated state.

> **Ejaculation**
> *The release of semen (sperm and fluids) from the penis during orgasm.*

Women have the potential of returning to an aroused state, but for men there is a refractory period in which they are unresponsive to sexual stimulation. This can last for minutes, hours, or longer depending on the man.

The Big "O"

Women are much more likely than men to have difficulty reaching orgasm during intercourse. In fact, one noted sex study found that only 30 to 50 percent of women experienced orgasm with straightforward intercourse. Does this mean that these women can't have an orgasm? No, it simply means that couples need to be more creative in their bedroom repertoire; clitoral stimulation is necessary for most women to reach orgasm.

Women can experience a variety of orgasms. A mild orgasm may cause three to five contractions, while an intense orgasm can have as many as twelve contractions. The intensity of a woman's (and man's) orgasm often changes from one

> **Multiple Orgasms**
> *More than one orgasm experienced within a relatively short period of time.*

sexual experience to another. Some women even have multiple orgasms.

The "Right" Amount of Sex

Many people wonder how often a "normal" couple has sex. The short answer is that there is no normal or right amount of sex. How much sex is right for a particular couple is determined by many factors and changes over the course of a relationship. There is certainly more sex during the "honeymoon" stage.

Other factors include the sexual clock of each partner, how busy they are, how many distractions they face (such as multiple jobs, conflicting job shifts, small children at home, and so on), and the aging process. There is wide variation, but the average for couples in their twenties is about twice a week, versus an average of twice a month for couples in their sixties (assuming an absence of sexual dysfunction).

But there is no reason for a couple to feel that they have to match any average. If a couple is happy having daily sex or once-a-year sex, then there is no problem. Problems only arise when one or both of the members of the couple are not content with the frequency. Masturbation is one option for the partner with the higher sexual desire.

Hormones Drive Libido

Hormones are a significant part of normal sexual function. Not only are they responsible for the physical differences between men and women and the ability to reproduce, but they also govern sexual thoughts and urges, genital arousal, and orgasm. Hormone levels vary daily, monthly, and also tend to decrease as we age.

Estrogen
Hormone produced by the ovaries that influences the development and maintenance of female sex organs and sexual characteristics such as breast development.

Estrogen is the primary female sex hormone. Although it does not have a direct effect on libido, it is necessary for vaginal lubrication and healthy vaginal tissue. When estrogen levels dip, a woman will have difficulty secreting lubrication and her thinning vaginal walls will be more susceptible to injury, pain, and even bleeding as a result of intercourse. For this reason (among others), some women opt for hormone replacement therapy (HRT) after menopause when estrogen levels drop considerably. Estrogen is also available in a topical cream.

Progesterone is another female hormone crucial for reproductive health. Progesterone prepares the lining of the uterus for implantation of a fertilized egg during the second half of the menstrual cycle. This hormone also promotes the development and health of the placenta during pregnancy. Progesterone is implicated in the occurrence of premenstrual syndrome.

HRT provides many benefits, including relief from many menopause symptoms, a boost in energy levels, alleviation of some forms of depression, protection against osteoporosis, and restoration of vaginal health, libido, and ability to orgasm. Some research indicates that HRT is even more effective in sexual improvement when used with testosterone. However, new research is emerging that there are also many risks associated with the use of HRT, such as an increase in breast cancer, heart attack, stroke, and blood clots. In fact, the largest study to date of HRT was recently disbanded because of the risks of HRT to women who still have their uterus (further research is still underway about the risks to women who have had hysterectomies). Given the latest - research, HRT is increasingly questioned as an appropriate treatment for women with a uterus. Its potential use should be carefully discussed with your health care provider.

The hormone testosterone, although primarily thought of as a male hormone, fuels the sex drive of both men and women. Abnormally low levels of testosterone ruins libido in both genders. Restoring testosterone levels in both men and women improves sexual desire and response, but its use for women is still controversial because there is such a delicate (and currently unknown) balance between how much testosterone is useful to a woman and how much has a masculinizing and damaging effect. The amount of testosterone given to women is much less than the amount given to men, since women normally have so much less of the hormone in their bodies. Several studies, particularly in postmenopausal women and women who have had their ovaries surgically removed, show that testosterone replacement therapy increases libido and sexual responsiveness. In women, testosterone is given in combination with estrogen. Increasing testosterone above average levels does not provide additional benefits, and in fact can lead to health problems.

Another hormone, called DHEA (which is shorthand for the long chemical name dehydroepiandrosterone) is produced by the adrenal glands. As discussed in Chapter 2, DHEA is the building block of many other sex-related hormones, including estrogen, testosterone, and progesterone. DHEA has also been linked to the production of pheromones (the scent chemicals that attract the opposite sex). In men and women, as DHEA levels fall with the passage of time, sex drive and sexual function suffer. DHEA is available as a dietary supplement, and some research indicates a benefit from its use. DHEA supplementation has been studied in men and women and generally found to have a boosting effect on libido. When women with sexual dysfunctions (both premenopausal and postmenopausal) were treated with DHEA, results were also promising. DHEA is generally used in the amount of 10–50 mg per day. However, there are cautions to consider, such as a potential raising of cholesterol levels, liver damage, and an increased risk of certain types of cancer. It is best to work with a nutrition-minded doctor while using DHEA.

TABLE 4.1. What Goes Wrong

	Men (% of population)	Women (% of population)
Sexual dysfunction (any type)	31–60	43–76
Low libido	15	30
Pain during intercourse	<5	10–15
Erectile dysfunction (mild, moderate, or severe)	31–52	
Premature ejaculation	30	
Sexual arousal disorder		10–20
Difficulty achieving orgasm		10–15

Men's Sex Concerns

Erectile dysfunction gets the most attention of the sexual dysfunctions that can affect men. So major a concern is ED that this book devotes an entire chapter to the problem; see Chapter 6.

Premature ejaculation is a concern of some men. With premature ejaculation, the male ejaculates very quickly after achieving an erection, sometimes even before penetration. This problem tends to be psychological, as opposed to physical, in nature. As such, consultation with a psychologist can be the most useful course of action. The psychologist will probably suggest some activities, such as the squeeze technique. There are also a handful of medications that may help; some are actually antidepressants that have been found to delay orgasm as a side effect. Talk to your doctor if you are interested in exploring this option.

Squeeze Technique
A method to treat premature ejaculation by applying pressure to the penis under the glans prior to orgasm in order to cause a partial loss of erection and delay orgasm.

A flagging libido is a concern of more than one in ten men. Decreased sex drive has numerous causes, including low testosterone levels, depression, fatigue, or as a side effect of certain medications (see the appendix for a list of the medications that can cause this).

Men who are able to get an erection but can't reach orgasm are generally treated by a psychologist, since this problem is primarily psychological in nature. It can, however, be related to physical causes. Diabetes can cause a loss of genital sensation as a result of nerve damage. The source of the problem can also be certain antidepressant medications.

Women's Sex Concerns

Women's sexual problems have not gotten the attention from the medical community that they merit. Unlike men—who, if they can't get an erection, simply can't have intercourse—women who are not sexually responsive can still have sex; it's just no fun. Over the years, many women brave enough to share their sexual frustrations with their doctors were merely told to use a lubricant. Or worse, their sexual health concerns were dismissed as either psychological or emotional problems. In actuality, the sexual problems of women (like men) are usually physical in nature, and these physical causes can be treated. Thankfully, in recent years the medical community has paid much better attention to this issue.

Loss of desire and other sexual problems in women are much more common than you might think, but it doesn't need to be this way. Most of these problems are treatable, whether psychological or physical in origin.

Four Types of Female Sexual Dysfunction

The first category of female sexual dysfunction is known as low sexual desire. A woman simply has a lack of interest in sex. Depression is a common cause of dampened libido. Certain medications (listed in the appendix), menopause, or low testosterone levels can also be to blame.

Second is sexual arousal disorder. In such cases, a woman lacks adequate vaginal lubrication and accompanying swelling of the external genitalia. Other aspects of arousal, such as nipple sensitivity, increased clitoral and labial sensation, and vaginal dilation, are generally impaired, as well. Female arousal, like male arousal, requires well-functioning circulation and nerve fibers. Smoking and cardiovascular disease are culprits here. If the problem is primarily inadequate lubrication for comfortable sex, use of topical lubricants can help.

The third category of problems facing women is difficulty or inability achieving orgasm. Some women have never had an orgasm, while others used to have orgasms, but after surgery, trauma, medication use, or hormone deficiency, no longer have them. Since most women reach orgasm as a result of clitoral stimulation (as opposed to just vaginal penetration)—and the clitoris is not directly stimulated during intercourse—the problem might easily be solved by providing the right type of stimulation (manual, oral, or with a vibrator directly to the clitoris). Before a woman assumes she has an orgasm disorder, she first should determine whether or not clitoral stimulation results in orgasm. If so, then the problem can be solved simply by changing sexual technique.

The final category is sexual pain disorders. When intercourse is painful a woman is said to suffer from dyspareunia. Numerous causes can account for this, and it is certainly a common problem. In one survey, 18 percent of healthy women reported experiencing frequent pain during intercourse. If the pain is at the vaginal entrance, the problem might be related to a local irritation as a result of spermicides or a yeast infection. Pain deeper in the vagina is commonly caused by the penis being inserted before the woman is fully aroused, which means that the vagina has not yet had a chance to expand. Endometriosis and fibroid tumors also account for some cases of dyspareunia.

Dyspareunia
Pain during intercourse, resulting from a yeast infection, a lack of sexual arousal, or a more serious health problem.

In some women the pain is related to a condition called vaginismus in which the lower third of the vagina has recurrent involuntary spasms. These spasms interfere with or even prevent intercourse. This is much less common than the other female sexual dysfunctions discussed in this section and is often triggered by past sexual trauma, such as sexual abuse, or painful intercourse that in turn causes the spasms in anticipation that future intercourse might also be painful. Vaginismus is generally treated with a two-pronged approach of psychological counseling and a procedure in which the woman uses a series of graduated dilators while focusing on the different sensations of muscle relaxation and contraction.

New Medical Treatment for Women

A new therapy for women with sexual dysfunction—the EROS-CTD (clitoral therapy device)—was approved by the Food and Drug Administration in May 2000. This device is placed over the clitoris and creates suction in order to increase blood flow and enhance clitoral engorgement. Studies have found that women experience increased sensation, better lubrication, improved ability to reach orgasm, and a greater overall satisfaction with sex after using the device. This device is a preferable choice for women who wish to avoid the potential side effects of pharmaceutical drugs.

The Bottom Line

To get the most out of your sex life, it's a good idea to understand the basics of sexual anatomy, and keep an eye on what could go wrong.

- Sexual responses are similar for men and women. The four stages are desire, arousal, orgasm, and resolution.

- Most women need clitoral stimulation in order to reach orgasm.

- Erectile dysfunction, premature ejaculation, and low libido are the most common sexual dysfunctions in men.

- For women, the most common sexual dysfunctions are low libido, sexual arousal disorder (the woman is interested, but her body doesn't respond), pain during intercourse, and difficulty achieving orgasm.

CHAPTER 5

CREATING INTIMACY

Maximizing your sexual health is not just about reconnecting with your passion, it's also about reconnecting with your partner. In the process of restoring or strengthening your intimacy, passion and sexual hunger for each other should naturally follow. Indeed, it becomes a circle in which greater intimacy leads to more and better sex, the sex in turn primes the feelings of intimacy, and so on.

More than Just a Pill

While Viagra has brought sexual dysfunction out of the closet and restored lost sex lives for many couples, the bottom line is that no pill—regardless of how effective it is—can by itself replace the loss of romance and affection that often surrounds sexual dysfunction. For example, a man experiencing erectile dysfunction for the first time feels confused and embarrassed, and, rather than discuss the issue with his partner, he is likely to withdraw emotionally and physically. This causes her to feel confused, rejected, and worry that she is no longer attractive to him. Years can go by without the problem being treated, and those years can do a lot of damage to a relationship. This damage needs to be addressed; simply popping a Viagra and expecting the sexual relationship to be perfect again will not work.

Regardless of whether or not a couple is trying to overcome a sexual dysfunction, it is important to recognize that men and women approach sex very differently. A man's body responds more quickly to sexual cues. This is compounded by the fact that many men feel desired and loved as a result of having sexual contact, while most women need to feel intimacy and emotional connection *before* their bodies will start to generate physical desire. This male/female mismatch has been at the root of many couples' downfall. Working together to find a balance that is fulfilling to both partners is vital to a relationship's success.

Stages of Intimate Relationships

Couples in a long-term relationship need to keep their expectations realistic. As fun and exhilarating as it is to fall in love, the fact is that this level of excitement is not possible to maintain. In fact, this initial infatuation stage—when a couple thinks of nothing but each other and the sex is thrilling and frequent—is not going to continue forever. As a relationship stabilizes, it moves into a phase of emotional attachment, where real love blooms. This represents a deeper level of commitment and also allows you to incorporate the relationship into the rest of your life; it is no longer all-consuming.

Infatuation
The early stage of a relationship, characterized by strong feelings of excitement and a powerful desire to be with a person; this state cannot last, but it can deepen into love.

Some couples mourn the loss of the infatuation stage, and this can lead to couple trouble. However, the most successful long-term relationships are the ones that maintain the attachment phase. These couples recognize that moving out of infatuation and into attachment does not mean falling out of love, it simply means that the relationship has matured. But by no means does this mean that sex can't still be great after many years of marriage. That's what this book is all about—finding ways to rediscover amorous adventures with your partner.

Couple Trouble

Relationship difficulties, such as emotional issues

and rejection by a partner, are fingered as the reason for failed marriages by 40 percent of women and 43 percent of men. Sexual difficulties usually go hand-in-hand with these problems. No aphrodisiac will be able to overcome sexual problems that are based in relationship conflict.

Many marriages turn into a business partnership of sorts, where housekeeping, finances, and social obligations shove intimacy to the back of the line. Poor communication, anger, a lack of trust, and a lack of connection are invariably factors here. These issues must be dealt with before sexual connection can be restored. If a couple has drifted so far apart that they cannot find their way back to intimacy on their own, a couple's counselor can help.

Intimacy Takes Work

If a couple's relationship problems seem relatively minor, the fixes might also be minor. For example, some couples keep the spark alive by making dates with each other to refocus some energy on intimacy. Spending time together, with no other distractions, can be the best way to rekindle a spark.

Intimacy takes input on your part, and paying attention to ways to please your partner is a great place to start. The next few sections will explain how sexually connecting with all five senses can reinvigorate a relationship.

Get in Touch

Of all the senses, touch contributes the most directly to sexual pleasure. Touch stimulates the release of oxytocin, one of the pleasure hormones. Oxytocin reaches peak levels at the point of orgasm, but it also contributes to a feeling of being bonded with your partner. Oxytocin is also released during the gentle touching of massage, hugging, and kissing.

Oxytocin
A hormone present during sexual excitement that encourages feelings of intimacy.

After the courting stage of a relationship has passed, many couples stop holding hands and may no longer touch at all in any affectionate ways other than intercourse. One or both partners can then end up feeling as though any touch that is initiated is simply a prelude to sex, and there's no real romance behind it. Touching each other—an arm around a shoulder, a hand resting on a thigh—at times that do not lead to sexual encounters helps build an overall closeness that in turn leads to more intimacy and better sex.

Partner massage is effective on many different levels. It stimulates the mind through increased concentration, stimulates the heart through a feeling of connection, and stimulates the body by virtue of touch. Massage is a wonderful way to show your love; it brings healing and pleasure at the same time. Here's how to give partner massage a try:

Step one: The tactile pleasure of hands on skin is enhanced by the use of oils. Choose an aromatherapy or massage oil. Choose scents that smell sensual to each partner. The essences most noted for their libido-enhancing qualities are ylang ylang, sandalwood, jasmine, clary sage, rose, bergamot, and cinnamon.

Step two: Set the mood by turning on soft music, unplugging the phone, and lighting candles. Candles are instant intimacy.

Step three: Pour the oil in your hands and rub your hands together to warm them before you begin to massage your partner. You can even warm your hands in a basin of hot water before you begin the massage.

Step four: Begin the massage as a G-rated experience, to establish a feeling of connection. Find out how soft or hard each partner likes to be massaged. This is a time for building anticipation. Work rhythmically with the strokes of the massage. Let your fingers follow the natural contours of your partner's body, gliding and caressing.

Step five: If it feels right to heat things up, move the massage into erogenous zones and enjoy where this experience takes you. Note, however, that not every massage need end up as sex; touch is a pleasant end in itself.

Understanding Yourself

In addition to indulging time touching your partner, it might be a good idea to spend some time getting to know your own body. Learning what type of touch (where, how much pressure, what type of rhythm) brings you pleasure and/or leads to orgasm will help you to communicate to your partner what experiences will be most satisfying. In general, women have more difficulty reaching orgasm, but both genders can benefit from this activity.

The Scent of Love

Scents have been recognized by every culture as an integral part of sexual experience. Fragrances are common parts of seduction, fertility rites, and marriage ceremonies in most cultures. Today's world, with its booming perfume and cologne businesses, is no exception. Explore the world of scents through scented candles, potpourri, incense, perfume, cologne, and/or scented massage oil.

Sexual attraction is also affected by smells we don't even realize are there: pheromones. Many sexual aspects of the lives of animals are governed by pheromones, and humans are not so different. In a pair of studies, one conducted with women and the other with men, synthesized pheromones were applied daily and sexual behaviors were tracked for a few months. In both studies, the men and women wearing pheromones noted significantly more sexual encounters (intercourse, kissing, petting, affection, and dates) than men and women given a fake spray. Clearly, pheromones act as an attractant to the opposite sex.

Pheromones
Faint chemical signals released from the skin that affect the mating rituals of much of the animal kingdom.

Food Fuels Passions

Food and sex, as we discussed in Chapter 1, often share an intimate bond. But besides the individual foods with reputations as aphrodisiacs, food in general often plays a big role during the seduction or courtship stage of a relationship. And it doesn't need to end there. Romantic dinners can continue to be a prelude to an evening of great sex. The food can even join you in the bedroom: Feeding each other or even eating erotic foods off each other's body are terrific ways to shake up the bedroom routine.

Setting the Mood

Setting a romantic mood often starts with selecting great music for the background. Music can ease the transition from a hectic day to an amorous evening by helping to relax and soothe the body. Many couples have certain types of music or individual songs that serve as cues that a romantic tryst is forthcoming.

Visual stimuli are very important in sexual arousal, especially for men. Some well-chosen items of lingerie can go a long way toward making the wearer feel sexy and in the mood while titillating the partner. Spending extra time during foreplay by slowly undressing each other is another sure way to heighten the mood. Maximizing visual excitement by doing such things as showering or bathing together, lounging in the buff, or even something as simple as keeping the lights on during lovemaking can all promote extra bedroom fireworks. In addition, eye contact is a powerful way for sexual partners to feel connected.

Assert Yourself

For both women and men, talking about sex in a personal way can be a scary endeavor—but it comes with great rewards. Revealing your sexual needs, desires, and wishes with your partner is much more effective than hoping your partner is a mind reader.

Before you start such an important conversation it is a good idea to spend some time beforehand organizing your thoughts. Next, make sure that your partner is in the mood to have such a talk; if he or she is distracted or tired, it's best to reschedule. Most important of all, make sure you emphasize the positive side of your sex life and relationship so that the conversation doesn't backfire. For example, instead of saying "Don't rub me so hard," say "I'd enjoy it much more if you stroked me gently."

Sexual assertiveness—knowing what you like and being open with your partner about it—makes a big difference, particularly in the sex lives of women. Sexually assertive women have been shown to have more sexual desire, more happiness with both their marriages and sex life, more frequent sex, and more orgasms.

Technique

Countless books have been written about sexual techniques; this book is not intended to replicate them. However, as an overview, a few ideas will be mentioned. Sexual fantasies are a common part of both men and women's sex lives. These fantasies serve a number of purposes, including an escape from bedroom boredom, a rehearsal for a new sexual experience you might want to try, and even a harmless exploration of scenarios that you don't really want to try but nonetheless find stimulating to imagine.

Touch is an essential part of sexual technique. The erogenous zones include not only the genitals, breasts, and lips, but also the buttocks, thighs, back of the neck, ears, hands, feet, and toes. Touching, stroking, and nibbling during foreplay are always arousing. Many couples find that manually stimulating the genitals or performing oral sex during foreplay or as the main event adds much variety and ex-

Erogenous Zones
The parts of the body most sensitive to erotic stimulation, especially the lips, breasts, and genitals.

citement to their sex lives. Exploring various sexual positions (again, there are many manuals that can be consulted on the topic) is another way for a couple to keep things fresh.

The Bottom Line

Intimacy is a powerful aphrodisiac in its own right. Strengthening the emotional connection with your partner results in a better bedroom relationship.

- Relationships go through different stages; the excitement of infatuation is replaced by deeper feelings of emotional attachment, otherwise known as love.

- Fizzling intimacy is a major culprit of failed marriages.

- Carving out time together to share a massage or linger over a romantic meal builds intimacy. However, more serious couple trouble will probably take a stronger fix—such as visits to a therapist.

- Being open and assertive about your sexual desires with your partner can bring more sexual satisfaction.

CHAPTER 6

ERECTILE DYSFUNCTION

Erectile dysfunction (ED) is defined as the inability to achieve or maintain an erection firm enough for intercourse. The condition profoundly affects quality of life and is associated with loss of self-esteem, poor self-image, depression, and increased tension with one's partner. The problem is more widespread than you may think: An estimated 31 to 52 percent of American men are or have been affected by some degree of erectile dysfunction. And about half of men over age forty will at some time face ED.

Types of Erectile Dysfunction

Erectile dysfunction is categorized as either primary or secondary. Primary erectile dysfunction is the term for men who have never been able to sustain a satisfactory erection, while men with secondary erectile dysfunction had normal erections at one point, but for some reason no longer do.

Erectile Dysfunction
The inability to maintain an erection, formerly known as impotence.

Furthermore, ED varies in its severity. Minimal dysfunction means that a man can usually keep an erection sufficient for intercourse; moderate dysfunction indicates only sometimes being able to achieve an erection capable of intercourse; and complete dysfunction means never being able to maintain an erection.

Causes of Erectile Dysfunction

It's been said that the penis is the divining rod of overall health, since most cases of erectile dysfunction are indicators of another disease. For this reason, it is very important to work with a doctor to pin down the underlying cause of ED and properly treat it.

The top cause of ED is cardiovascular disease. As discussed earlier, problems with blood flow in the body will have an obvious impact on erections, since erections are dependent on the penis becoming engorged with blood. Blockages in arteries are the worst culprit here, and these blockages can generally be traced back to high cholesterol levels, smoking, diabetes, or high blood pressure.

Diabetes is a big risk factor for developing erectile dysfunction. Aside from the blood flow problems already mentioned, diabetes can also damage the nerves necessary for firm erections. Men with diabetes tend to develop ED at an earlier age than nondiabetics. Some surveys have found ED in as many as 75 percent of diabetic men. These men can protect themselves by keeping their blood-sugar levels as normal as possible.

Diabetes
A disease characterized by too much sugar in the blood, which damages blood vessels.

Surgery or traumatic accidents to the pelvis can cause ED. It can also be caused as a side effect of a medication or can be related to depression or other psychological problems. Chapter 8 discusses all of the medical causes of erectile dysfunction in greater detail.

Psychological Versus Physical Source of Erectile Dysfunction

In years past, erectile dysfunction was believed to have a psychological source in 90 percent of cases, and a physical cause in the remaining 10 percent. Today those figures are completely reversed, with physical problems being implicated in nine out of ten men with ED. In reality, however, few cases are so clear-cut. For example, a man who is prescribed a new medication that unbeknownst to him has sexual side effects will likely become confused and depressed when he has trouble functioning in the bedroom. This psychological component can then impact the couple's relationship and, even if the medication is changed, he may continue to have anxiety and fear of failure when it comes to sex.

Virtually all healthy men experience several erections during the REM phase of sleep. Thus, determining whether or not a man has sleep erections can help determine whether his erectile dysfunction is physical or psychological. Presumably, a man who is physically capable of an erection during sleep should be capable of an erection while awake. There are sleep labs where this is tested, as well as a gauge men can put on their penis at home.

REM Sleep
Active sleep (as opposed to nonactive, deep sleep) when dreaming occurs, the heartbeat accelerates, blood pressure rises, and muscles twitch.

Older Men More at Risk

Erectile dysfunction is not an inevitable consequence of aging, although it does become more prevalent as the years go by. The Massachusetts Male Aging Study, the most comprehensive study of ED, found that while only 5 percent of men in their forties experience complete erectile dysfunction (that is, they never are able to sustain an erection sufficient for intercourse), by the time a man is in his seventies, the numbers have tripled to 15 percent. Likewise, in the process of aging from forty to seventy, the likelihood of having a moderate case of ED doubles from 17 to 34 percent. In all, more than half of adult men report having at least one episode of erectile dysfunction.

Herbal Remedies

As discussed in Chapter 2, several natural remedies have proved successful in restoring erections to a significant number of men. Keep in mind, however, that the herbs and supplements discussed here are not meant to be taken together at the same time.

After reading about the individual supplements, choose one to try.

Yohimbe is probably the best-known herb for erectile dysfunction. The bark of the yohimbe tree contains a compound called yohimbine that increases blood vessel dilation, improving erections. A prescription medication of yohimbine is also available.

A double-blind, placebo-controlled study put yohimbe to the test by comparing the effects of yohimbine (up to 30 mg per day) in men who had erectile dysfunction and normally functioning men. The yohimbe supplements resulted in "strong positive effects" for 27 percent of the men with ED.

It's best to start out with small amounts of yohimbine, since this herb is associated with potentially adverse effects. Yohimbine in amounts greater than 40 mg daily can cause chills, vertigo, muscle weakness, high blood pressure, or prolonged, painful erections. In addition, anyone taking yohimbe should avoid foods rich in tyramine (which include cheese, red wine, and liver), since this combination can theoretically cause dangerously high blood pressure.

Ginkgo has a well-known reputation for promoting circulation to the blood vessels that feed the brain, but the same mechanism of action also boosts blood flow to the penis. A preliminary trial of sixty men with erectile dysfunction due to circulation problems reported that 60 mg per day of ginkgo extract for at least a year resulted in restored virility in half of the men. (See Chapter 2 for cautions when using ginkgo.)

Ginseng has long been associated with male potency, and now experts might understand why. Blood flow in the body is regulated by nitric oxide; thus, the ability of a man to have an erection depends, in part, on nitric oxide. Ginseng has been found to enhance the synthesis of nitric oxide. A study of ninety men with erectile dysfunction found that, compared to placebo or a drug (trazodone), ginseng resulted in significantly greater sexual desire and erectile function.

The amino acid arginine also raises nitric oxide levels and can help men with erectile dysfunction. The herbs muira puama and tribulus both long have been believed to improve erections. Kava is a relaxing herb, so if anxiety is the source of erectile dysfunction, this herb can help. All these herbs and supplements are discussed in more detail in Chapter 2.

What Your Doctor Might Suggest

Tragically, more than 80 percent of men with erectile dysfunction simply ignore the problem and don't seek treatment. However, ED is almost always treatable, by one method or another. So if you decide natural remedies are not for you and you make a doctor's appointment, here's what your doctor will likely suggest.

The oral medication Viagra has quickly become the first-line treatment for erectile dysfunction, partly because it has the highest acceptance rate among men. (Two new medications in the same family as Viagra, called vardenafil and Cialis, are poised to enter the market this year, pending FDA approval. They work faster and last longer than Viagra and may have fewer side effects.) Viagra is far less invasive and cumbersome than the other leading medical techniques for ED, as you will see. Even so, there are problems associated with its use, which will be discussed later in this chapter.

Intracavemous injection is extremely effective, but because it involves injecting a needle into the penis, few men choose it. Prostaglandin E1 (PGE1) is often the medication injected into the penis, although various combinations of PGE1 with papaverine and phentolamine can be used.

Intracavemous Injection
A procedure that uses a small needle to inject erection-promoting drugs directly into the penile tissue.

A man choosing this option goes through several sessions with his doctor to determine the best amount and combination of medication. The man then learns how to inject the medication himself. The tiny insulin needle is almost painless to use. It takes about fifteen minutes of stimulation to achieve an erection. The erection then lasts about an hour. This treatment can only be used twice per week. Potential problems with its use, aside from needle squeamishness, are prolonged erections that last hours, bruises at the injection site, and painful erections.

A vacuum constriction device is a plastic cylinder attached by a tube to a pump that "draws" blood into the penis by reverse pressure to cause an erection. The pumping can take five minutes to achieve an erection firm enough for penetration. The erection is maintained by placing a tight elastic band or ring around the base of the penis. About 80 percent of men using this treatment are satisfied with their erections and ability to have intercourse. However, the band can only be kept in place for thirty minutes, after which the penis can become painful.

Urethral suppositories induce an erection by delivering medications directly into the urethra. The process is simple and relatively comfortable. There are some problems with its use, including mild pain in the penis, vaginal burning or itching in the partner, dizziness, and prolonged erections.

A last-resort option is a penile prosthesis. Semi-rigid silicone rods are one option; they are surgically implanted into the penis. This procedure is irreversible because the erectile tissue is damaged during the surgery. The main disadvantage is that a man will have the equivalent of an erection at all times, not just when he wants to have sex. A better option is an inflatable cylindrical implant that is connected to a reservoir implanted in the lower pelvis. A pump in the scrotum is then used to inflate or deflate the penis.

Viagra: A "Happy Accident"

The discovery of Viagra was actually a happy accident. This drug, generic name sildenafil, was known to dilate blood vessels and for this reason was being researched in Great Britain in the 1980s as a treatment for coronary heart disease. It failed as a heart medication, but when the research trial was discontinued, the researchers weren't ready to give up on sildenafil, because many of the men in the study reported having improved erections. Remember, cardiovascular diseases are a major cause of ED because the blood vessels feeding the penis don't convey enough blood for an erection. So these cardiac patients also had a high rate of erectile dysfunction. While the Viagra didn't end up helping their hearts, it jump-started the blood flow to their genitals and led to an unexpected sexual rejuvenation.

Viagra's manufacturer (Pfizer) soon followed up on the reports of these men's renewed sexual vigor with a series of double-blind, placebo-controlled studies conducted specifically on men with erectile dysfunction. This series of studies, twenty-one in all, found that about four out of five men responded well to Viagra, compared to one in four men taking the dummy pills.

Viagra works by blocking activity of an enzyme called PDE5. PDE5's role is to end an erection (theoretically, after successful intercourse) by breaking down the enzymes responsible for relaxing muscle tissue and allowing increased blood flow to the penis. When PDE5 is prevented from doing this, erections improve. Because Viagra doesn't have any effect on the compounds that *produce* erections (only on those that end them), it won't trigger an erection without the presence of sexual stimulation, which is another advantage over other medical treatments; it simply allows (in many cases) the male machinery to respond to stimuli.

PDE5
An enzyme, found primarily in the penis, responsible for ending an erection by breaking down the erection-producing enzymes present in the tissue.

More than one million prescriptions per month were written for Viagra when it first hit the market, making it the most successfully released drug in the history of medicine. Currently about ten million men have used Viagra. Clearly, there were a lot of men in need of help with their erectile dysfunction.

Advantages and Disadvantages of Viagra

One of the best things about Viagra is that it helped remove some of the taboo from a difficult subject. Erectile dysfunction quickly went from a topic no one would discuss to one that Bob Dole filmed commercials about. For the first time, vast numbers of men were willing to talk with their doctors about their sexual health and lack of sexual satisfaction. As we have seen in this chapter, Viagra was also a welcome departure from the cumbersome treatments that preceded it, which tended to remove the spontaneity from sex, at best, or lead to painful and dangerous side effects, at worst. While Viagra has not solved all of these problems completely, it is certainly a major step forward.

But there is a less obvious down side to Viagra. Viagra is an easy fix—what could be simpler than popping a pill—and easy fixes are not necessarily the best ways to deal with erectile dysfunction. The penis is designed to have erections; if that is not happening then it's a sign of bigger problems in the body. Instead of just popping a Viagra and ignoring the message, you should explore the underlying cause of the erectile dysfunction. If the cause is diabetes, cardiovascular disease, or another health problem, you'll be glad you didn't ignore it.

Of course, another big problem with using Viagra is that it is linked to an ever-growing list of side effects and problems. In fact, there are hundreds of deaths that have been associated with Viagra in some way. This is why the natural treatments for ED discussed in this chapter are so important—though even with natural treatments, it is essential to heed all warnings.

Viagra absolutely cannot be taken by anyone using nitrate drugs in any form; a catastrophic collapse in blood pressure can result. There are over one hundred drugs on the market that contain nitrates; please check carefully if you think you might be taking one. Side effects from Viagra can include headache, facial flushing, upset stomach, and a severe drop in blood pressure. One quirky side effect from Viagra can be a temporary colorblindness of the colors blue and green, caused because the retina contains an enzyme called PDE6 that is closely related to PDE5 and is also affected by Viagra. The effect is harmless and goes away after a few hours.

Nitrate Drugs
A family of drugs often used by those with angina and high blood pressure.

Does Viagra Work for Women?

Because sexual arousal in women depends on similar physiological processes to those that occur in men, such as increased blood flow to the genitals, many people wondered if Viagra could help women as well. This curiosity resulted in several double-blind, placebo-controlled studies of women. The results showed benefits for women in line with those seen in sexually dysfunctional men. Women of all ages with sexual dysfunctions (lagging libido, decreased lubrication, low arousal, or difficulty achieving orgasm) have taken Viagra and achieved more frequent sexual fantasies, more sex, and more enjoyable sex. Clearly, Viagra is not just for men and many doctors are now prescribing Viagra for women experiencing sexual dysfunction.

The Bottom Line

As many as half of all men will, at times, deal with erectile dysfunction.

- Heart disease, diabetes, depression, and medication side effects are all major causes of erectile dysfunction.

- Only 10 percent of erectile dysfunction is traced to a psychological cause.

- Dietary supplement remedies for erectile dysfunction include the herbs yohimbe, ginkgo, and ginseng, and the amino acid arginine.

- Conventional medical treatments for erectile dysfunction include Viagra, intracavemous injections, vacuum constriction devices, urethral suppositories, and penile prosthetics.

CHAPTER 7

INFERTILITY

The primary subject of this book is achieving a healthy and supremely satisfying sex life, but it is easy to forget that sometimes the goal of sex is more than simple pleasure and bedroom gymnastics. When the goal is conception, even the most mind-blowing sex can be ultimately unsatisfactory if that goal isn't met. Infertility can be emotionally devastating to a couple, so no book on sexual health would be complete without a chapter on the subject.

Very Treatable Problem

One out of ten Americans of reproductive age is affected by infertility, which is defined as the inability to achieve pregnancy after at least one year of unprotected intercourse. Millions of dollars are spent every year by couples in search of a diagnosis and treatment for their fertility problems. The cause of infertility can generally be determined in 85 percent of cases, with the responsibility evenly divided between the man and woman. The good news is that modern medicine can help infertile couples become pregnant in about 60 percent of cases.

The First Year: Waiting and Charting

Unless there is a known health problem, most doctors will have a couple try to get pregnant for one year before suggesting medical intervention. While waiting, however, a woman should chart her menstrual cycle. This serves two purposes. It reveals the best time to have intercourse, and it can indicate if there is a potential problem with ovulation, which

Ovulation
The monthly release of an egg from a woman's ovary.

would save the couple from unnecessarily waiting an entire year before taking further action. (A cycle that has fewer than twenty-five days or more than thirty-five days can indicate that ovulation is not occurring.)

One simple way to determine if you are ovulating is by taking a daily basal temperature (your temperature when you first wake up in the morning) for one or more months. Using a basal body thermometer, which is more accurate at detecting minute changes to body temperature than is a standard thermometer, you take your temperature every morning before getting out of bed. You should notice a sharp rise in temperature right before ovulation. The temperature stays at this elevated point until your period starts. Couples trying to get pregnant should have sex at least twice during the three or four days before and after the rise in temperature. More frequent sex is not necessarily better, since it can decrease the man's sperm count, making conception less likely.

Another sign that ovulation is imminent is an increase in quantity of vaginal mucus. This mucus should be thinner than usual and very stretchy, almost like the uncooked white part of an egg. There are also ovulation predictor kits available on the market.

Time to See Your Doctor

A visit to the doctor to discuss possible infertility problems will start with an interview of both partners and a general physical exam of the woman, including a Pap smear. The interview is very important; everything from the woman's menstrual cycle to thyroid problems, abortions, abdominal surgery, both partners' history with sexually transmitted diseases, and other related health conditions will be discussed and identified as potential sources of the fertility problem.

Although men and women are equally likely to be the source of infertility, the next step focuses on the man, since this is easier, less expensive, and less invasive. Diagnosing male infertility starts with a sperm count. The man brings a room-temperature semen sample in a sterile plastic cup to his doctor, who examines it under a microscope for living sperm. Numerous things can affect sperm count, including alcohol, drugs, cigarettes, and medical conditions.

Pap Smear
A test in which cells from the cervix are scraped away to be examined for abnormalities.

Investigating the Woman's Fertility

If the man's sperm appears to be healthy, then the medical workup moves on to the woman's reproductive health. A thorough patient history and certain diagnostic tests are necessary. As discussed earlier in this chapter, a common cause of female infertility is anovulation, or lack of ovulation. Several prescription medications are available to induce ovulation.

Another common cause of female infertility is damage to the fallopian tubes, often from endometriosis, infection, or past ectopic pregnancy. Either the sperm cannot reach the egg because of a blockage in the tubes, or the fertilized egg cannot reach the uterus for implantation. This type of problem is diagnosed with a test called a hysterosalpingogram (HSG), in which dye is used to make the uterus and fallopian tubes visible in an x-ray. Surgery is sometimes recommended to repair damaged tubes; other couples opt for in vitro fertilization.

Endometriosis
A health problem in which cells that normally line the uterus grow elsewhere in the pelvic cavity, causing heavy periods, pain, and an increased risk of infertility.

Although less likely than the first two problems discussed, some women's infertility is traced to problems with the cervix. The cervix can produce either too little mucus or mucus that is incompatible with the sperm's survival. Sometimes the cervix has extensive scarring (from infection, childbirth, or surgery) that prevents sperm from passing through. Bringing your doctor a sample of cervical mucus taken after intercourse can clarify the problem. If the sperm in the mucus are not swimming well, then the mucous environment might be the issue. If this is the source of infertility, your doctor may suggest taking low-dose estrogen (oral or topical form) to improve the cervical mucus. If the cervix is not allowing the passage of sperm, a doctor can use a procedure to introduce the sperm directly into the uterus.

Finally, some women have a luteal phase defect. The luteal phase of the menstrual cycle is the part of the cycle after ovulation. It generally lasts fourteen days, and during this time the hormone progesterone is responsible for preparing the uterine lining for implantation of a fertilized egg. If the ovaries do not secrete enough progesterone, implantation may not be able to take place. In such cases, progesterone (in the form of oral or vaginal suppositories) might be prescribed.

Treating the Problem Naturally

A basic multivitamin and mineral supplement is a good place to start for a woman trying to conceive. One recent study tracked the fertility effect of a multivitamin supplement compared to a placebo in almost 8,000 women. Women taking the supplements achieved pregnancy in fewer menstrual cycles, which translated to a 5 percent increase in fertility. Interestingly, the number of twins and other multiple births also slightly increased as a result of the supplement regimen.

What's behind this result? Several nutrients play key roles in women's reproductive health. Deficiencies of iron and the B vitamins interfere with normal fertility. Iron deficiency is very common in women; in fact, an estimated 7.8 million American women are iron-deficient. A woman experiencing infertility problems should work with a physician to determine her iron levels; many infertile women have conceived after restocking their iron stores.

Animal research shows that a deficiency of vitamin E can also produce infertility. In people, one study found that fertility improved when supplements providing 100–200 IU of vitamin E were taken by both members of the infertile couple.

Another nutrient to consider is PABA (para-aminobenzoic acid), which is a substance in the B-complex family. Many years ago, an interesting study suggested that PABA supplements increase the pregnancy rate in infertile women, possibly by influencing hormone levels. However, follow-up research to confirm this association remains to be done.

Supplements for Baby-Minded Men

A common cause of male infertility is poor sperm quality (insufficient number of sperm or poor sperm motility). Several nutrients, including vitamin C, zinc, and vitamin E, play a role in the production of healthy sperm. Vitamin C is crucial. As an antioxidant, it protects sperm from free radical damage—a function that is particularly important for smokers. Vitamin C also helps treat one cause of male infertility, a condition called sperm agglutination. Men with this condition show improved fertility after increasing their vitamin C intake.

Sperm Agglutination
A condition in which sperm stick together and for this reason are not able to properly swim to find an egg.

Vitamin B_{12} may help infertile men, but studies with this nutrient have used injections of vitamin B_{12}, which must be provided by a physician. Coenzyme Q_{10} has also been found to improve sperm production in some men.

Another nutrient strongly linked to male fertility is zinc. When zinc intake and markers of fertility in men were assessed in one study, the men with a low-zinc intake (1.4 mg daily), compared to the high-intake group (10.4 mg daily), showed adverse effects in their serum testosterone levels, volume of semen, and amount of zinc lost in the semen.

Improved intake of certain amino acids can also

be useful for infertile men. Arginine is needed to make sperm, and research shows that several months of arginine supplementation increases sperm count and improves sperm quality. Carnitine has also been found to help men with low sperm counts. Carnitine is readily found in meat and dairy products and is also available as a dietary supplement.

A carotenoid called lycopene, which is most plentiful in tomatoes, might aid male fertility. When men with fertility problems were given supplements of lycopene for three months, 36 percent of the couples reported the good news of a positive pregnancy test over the next nine months.

The Bottom Line

Infertility is an increasingly common problem, but fortunately it is also increasingly treatable.

- A basal body thermometer can be used daily to determine when ovulation takes place; ovulation predictor kits are also available.

- A doctor might conduct one or more tests in either or both members of a couple to determine the source of infertility. Common causes include endometriosis, inhospitable cervical mucus, or inadequate hormone production.

- Supplements for women with infertility to consider include a multivitamin/mineral, iron, B vitamins, vitamin E, and PABA.

- Male fertility-boosting supplements include vitamin C, zinc, vitamin E, vitamin B_{12}, arginine, carnitine, and lycopene.

CHAPTER 8

TALK TO
YOUR DOCTOR

There are many medical causes of sexual dysfunction—including depression, cardiovascular disease, diabetes, other medications, and surgery of the reproductive organs—most of which have been touched on briefly in various parts of this book. However, this chapter will delve more deeply into the potential for sexual dysfunction triggered by these health problems.

Not in the Mood

Being "in the mood" is a whole lot less likely if you're in a bad mood. This is common sense, but if you doubt it, a handful of studies have measured sexual response during positive and negative moods. No big surprises here: Being in a good mood is more conducive to feeling sexually aroused.

In their extreme form, mood problems can end up as full-blown depression. Depression can be caused by a chemical imbalance in the brain, severe stress, grief, emotional conflict, or a combination of these factors. Depression is widespread, especially for women.

Depression
A serious health problem manifesting as an overwhelming feeling of sadness and inability to function normally.

Twice as many women as men suffer from depression, with about 20 percent of women developing depression some time in their lives.

Depression will certainly put a serious damper on sexual desire—as well as many other aspects of life—and it needs to be treated before learning whether there are other causes of the sexual dysfunction. In many cases, resolving the depression takes care of the sexual problem. Ironically, many antidepressant medications have sexual side effects. The herb St. John's wort is a natural treatment for mild cases of depression. One of its main advantages is that it has no sexual side effects. The standard recommendation is 300 mg of St. John's wort extract taken three times per day. Some people experience sensitivity to sunlight when taking this herb. In addition, it should not be taken by those using antidepressants in the class of selective serotonin reuptake inhibitors (SSRIs). There are also some "sex-friendly" antidepressants, such as Wellbutrin (bupropion), that have much less effect on sexual function. See the appendix for a list of medications known to have sexual side effects.

Unhealthy Heart, Unhealthy Genitals

Atherosclerosis causes a buildup of fatty material known as plaque on the walls of arteries. Well known for cutting off blood flow to the heart or brain, causing a heart attack or stroke, atherosclerosis can also affect blood vessels elsewhere in the body. Atherosclerosis is generally linked to high cholesterol levels, diabetes, hypertension (high blood pressure), and/or cigarette smoking.

Atherosclerosis
Hardening of the arteries, a progressive form of cardiovascular disease characterized by buildup of plaque in artery walls.

During an erection, the small arteries that feed blood into the penis dilate in size from five to ten times in diameter. If these arteries have a buildup of plaque that blocks the vessel by 15 percent or more, there will be adverse effects on the quality of erection, or even the ability to achieve an erection. This blockage is the number one cause of erectile dysfunction in cases that do not have a psychological component. Not only can ED be a sign that cardiovascular disease is present, it can also be a marker for how the disease is progressing. As the erectile dysfunction worsens, it is likely that overall cardiovascular health is in jeopardy. In women, the same buildup of plaque can reduce blood flow to the genitals and interfere with the ability to become aroused.

High blood pressure is a potential problem in both men and women because it can damage the blood vessels, making them more prone to plaque buildup. In addition, as discussed later in this chapter, many of the medications used to treat high blood pressure can also cause sexual dysfunction.

Heart Attacks During Sex

Many people who have had a heart attack are fearful that having sex will trigger another attack. This risk is actually quite low. In a healthy middle-aged man or woman, the chance of having a heart attack during intercourse is about two chances per million for each hour of sexual intercourse. For an adult suffering from heart disease, the numbers only go up to twenty chances per million for each hour of sex.

Of course, you should talk to your doctor about any concerns and follow the doctor's advice, but in general, most people can resume sexual intercourse three to four months after a heart attack. For people who have had a stroke, it is very unlikely that sexual exertion will cause another stroke.

Diabetes

Diabetes can have a big impact on sexuality. Between 30 and 70 percent of diabetic men are affected by erectile dysfunction, since diabetes often damages the peripheral nervous system. Diabetes-related nerve damage can also interfere with female arousal and orgasm.

Peripheral Nervous System
The network of nerves branching out from the spinal cord to all parts of the body.

Male Pelvic Surgery or Trauma

Any pelvic surgery or trauma that damages the blood and nerve supply to the pelvic region is a potential cause of erectile dysfunction. Prostate cancer surgery all too often injures pelvic nerves and in this way results in ED. Fortunately, recent advances in this surgery have greatly reduced the number of men left with this unfortunate side effect. However, the location of the cancer determines how the surgery will need to proceed, and many men are not eligible for the nerve-sparing procedure. Thus, depending on the type of surgery needed, the incidence of ED following prostate cancer surgery varies from a low of 15 percent to a disheartening high of 60 to 85 percent.

Prostate Gland
The gland located below the bladder and surrounding the urethra. Prostate fluids assist reproduction by improving the survival time of sperm.

Interference of the Enlarged Prostate Gland

Noncancerous enlargement of the prostate gland, known as benign prostatic hyperplasia (BPH), will be experienced by more than half of all men over the age of fifty, and 80 percent of men ages eighty and older. Unfortunately, as the prostate enlarges, it can clamp down on the urethra and interfere with urination. Men with BPH need to urinate more frequently, may have difficulty starting the stream, have less force, dribble at the end, or need to get up several times a night to go to the bathroom. Advanced BPH can also soften erections, dampen libido, and interfere with sexual performance.

BPH
Benign prostatic hyperplasia, an enlargement of the prostate gland not associated with cancer but leading to urinary difficulty.

The good news is that your doctor can prescribe a fairly effective drug called Proscar (finasteride), but the bad news is that this drug can cause the side effects of erectile dysfunction and loss of libido in 5 percent of men. Natural remedies can often accomplish the same goal without the sexual interference.

Saw palmetto is the leading herb in this area. Saw palmetto has been shown to be superior to placebo and comparable to Proscar for improving urine flow rates and residual urine. Saw palmetto is believed to inhibit an enzyme that otherwise would convert testosterone to a more active form, which in turn aggravates BPH. Thus, this herb minimizes the inflammation that is problematic in BPH. Saw palmetto is recommended for early-stage BPH. Many herbalist recommend saw palmetto extracts that contain a fat-soluble or "liposterolic" portion of the herb in the amount of 320 mg per day of the liposterolic herbal extract. Best of all, saw palmetto has a very good safety profile, so it is a great choice for almost any man with BPH. Please note, however, that it may take numerous weeks of use before saw palmetto shows positive results.

An herb call pygeum is another option. When a group of men who had erectile dysfunction, in addition to either BPH or prostatitis (inflammation of the prostate), took supplements of pygeum, not only did the pygeum help their BPH or prostatitis, it also improved sexual function and their ability to have erections. Side effects with pygeum are rare; the standard dose is 50–100 mg taken twice a day. Stinging nettles are another potential remedy for BPH. Stinging nettles work in a similar manner to saw palmetto and pygeum to reduce inflammation in the prostate and these three herbs are often used in combination for BPH. Supplements of freeze-dried stinging nettles are generally used in the amount of 300–500 mg several times per day.

Pollen extract has been used with success in Europe for BPH for almost half a century. According to the handful of studies conducted with pollen extract, it aids BPH through an anti-inflammatory action that helps the bladder contract and pass urine, as well as relaxing the urethra to facilitate the passing of urine. The only pollen extract on the market is named Cernilton; fortunately, it's the one used in the tests. No side effects have been reported with the use of pollen extract, however, there is a theoretical risk that a person with severe hay fever could experience allergy symptoms. Cernilton is generally used in the amount of 60–120 mg taken three times per day.

Female Pelvic Surgery

Pelvic surgery of any kind has the potential to damage the nerves and blood vessels necessary for proper function of the vagina, uterus, and clitoris. Damage can then interfere with sexual sensation and the arousal process. Avoiding nerves and blood vessels during surgery is impossible, since the location of all the nerves and blood vessels of the female body simply hasn't been mapped out yet.

Hysterectomy is one of the most common pelvic operations, with about 600,000 hysterectomies performed each year. There are conflicting reports as to whether sexuality is positively or negatively affected by hysterectomy. For some women, sex gets better, because the health problems that necessitated the hysterectomy (such as uterine fibroids, endometriosis, or other painful conditions) are now gone. But for others, the operation can leave them with difficulties reaching sexual arousal and orgasm. If the hysterectomy removed the ovaries, then hormone levels are drastically altered, with a corresponding effect on libido.

Hysterectomy
The surgical removal of the uterus and sometimes the ovaries and cervix, as well.

Other Medical Causes of Sexual Dysfunction

Thyroid conditions (both hypothyroidism and hyperthyroidism) can be associated with erectile dysfunction. Peyronie's disease is characterized by a curvature of the penis, caused by scar tissue in the penis. In severe cases, this can interfere with or even prevent intercourse. Damage to the nervous system of the brain, from Parkinson's, stroke, Alzheimer's, brain tumors, or trauma (such as spinal cord injuries), can also interfere with the electrical messages needed for normal erections and female sexual response.

Yeast infections and urinary tract infections can indirectly interfere with sexual function in women, since the discomfort of the condition makes sex uncomfortable. Sex should be avoided during the time the infection is being treated.

Men, Sex, and Getting Older

As the years go by, men experience a gradual increase in the length of the refractory phase of sex. In a healthy twenty-year-old, the refractory phase may only last five minutes. A man in his forties might need up to an hour before a second erection is possible, and the average sixty-year-old probably would be out of commission until the next day.

Refractory Phase
The time just after an orgasm in which no amount of sexual stimulation will lead to an erection.

Getting older also tends to increase the amount of stimulation a man needs to get an erection in the first place. While a twenty-year-old needs virtually no stimulation to be aroused and is exceedingly likely to ejaculate during a sexual encounter (although it may be difficult for him to control the timing of the ejaculation), an older man needs much more direct stimulation to achieve an erection, and even so, the erection is probably not as hard as it was in younger years. The older man, however, has much more control over when he ejaculates. While the intensity of orgasm is often reported as less than it was in younger years, older men do report that their orgasms are more prolonged.

Hormone production also slows down with advancing age. The lower levels of testosterone seen in sixty-year-old men are accompanied by reduced virility, less muscle mass, loss of strength, a lower libido, and erectile dysfunction. The equivalent of menopause in women, this hormone change is coming to be known as andropause. Low testos-

Andropause
A decline in hormone levels experienced by older men that is analogous to menopause in women and results in several physical and sexual changes.

terone is the hallmark of andropause, and some doctors are now recommending that such men be treated with testosterone replacement therapy.

Although the aging process affects male fertility less than female fertility, there is still a decline as time goes by. Sperm production declines with each passing year. Even so, only about 50 percent of men are infertile by age eighty or older. The ability to maintain erections does not fare as well. Erectile dysfunction is increasingly common as men age.

Women, Sex, and Stages of Life

Research tracking women's libido during different stages of the menstrual cycle has been conflicting. No clear change in libido or arousal ability appears at different times of the month. Many women take birth control pills during their reproductive years. In many cases, sex is more enjoyable for the women since the fear of pregnancy is removed, but some women report a loss of libido and vaginal dryness due to the hormones in the pill. This is more common in progestin-dominant pills such as Modicon, Brevicon, or Ovcon.

Pregnancy can also affect sex drive. In general, women have decreased desire in the first trimester, increased desire in the second trimester, and decreased again in the third trimester. Not surprisingly, sexual interludes are lower than average for a couple after a baby arrives, most likely due to sleep deprivation and lack of free time.

Although vaginal lubrication might take longer to achieve, there is some good sexual news for women as they get older. Many women find sex in their middle years to be better than ever. They've learned what pleases them and are better about vocalizing it. It also helps that at this stage children are less of a drain on energy levels and may even be grown and out of the house. At long last, the time and attention is available to devote to regular sex.

Other women have a different experience at this age. They might be single for the first time in decades, as a result of divorce or the death of a spouse. Starting over in a new relationship can be exciting, but unsettling. Many women are insecure about their bodies as they change with the passage of time. An even bigger problem with the sex lives of this age group is that many of their male partners are reaching the prime age for experiencing sexual dysfunction themselves, or having a health condition that necessitates using a medication with sexual side effects. The woman may be ready, willing, and able, but her partner might not be up to the job.

Menopause and Beyond

As women reach later middle age, their sex lives often go to pot. There are many reasons for this, including the physical changes of menopause, simply getting older, and the increasing likelihood that their partners have developed a sexual dysfunction. Hormone replacement therapy (especially when androgens are included in the formula) can go far to counteract the physical problems associated with menopause. But their use comes with risk, and whether or not to use hormone replacement therapy is a decision each woman should consider carefully and discuss with her health care provider. The latest evidence shows that use of HRT by women who still have a uterus is associated with a higher risk of breast cancer, heart attack, stroke, and blood clots.

Hot flashes are the classic sign of menopause, but there are many other physical changes associated with this change of life. The vagina and labia have a large number of estrogen receptors and are very sensitive to changes in estrogen levels. As estrogen levels drop during and after menopause, many women experience decreased vaginal lubrication and thinning of the vagina walls. When this occurs, the resulting pain during intercourse can interfere with libido. Estrogen replacement therapy (pills, patch, or vaginal cream) can counteract this somewhat, but it also comes with side effects. Other options include over-the-counter products that are inserted vaginally a few times a week to maintain vaginal moisture, or simply using lubrication prior to intercourse.

The herb black cohosh has been used by many women with good success in controlling some of the uncomfortable symptoms of menopause, particularly hot flashes. Standardized extracts of the herb are available and generally taken in the amount of 20–40 mg twice daily. Black cohosh is not associated with any side effects when used in this amount.

Ironically, an active sex life in the postmenopausal years is good for the libido and the sexual organs, keeping the vaginal tissue healthy and moist and delaying the aging process. Women who continue to be sexually active through menopause and beyond retain a higher level of sexual desire.

Is Your Problem in Your Medicine Chest?

As this book has mentioned, drugs, both prescription and over-the-counter, can have a big impact on sexual health. They can interfere with blood flow to the genitals, contribute to vaginal dryness, dampen libido, and alter hormones involved in the sexual response. It is important to consult a physician to rule these out as the source of any sexual problems. All too many people have discovered that they traded in one health problem for another with a new medication—that is, their initial health complaint was resolved but now they face sexual dysfunction. In many cases there are drug or treatment alternatives that treat the initial problem without the specter of sexual side effects.

Many drugs chemically crush the libido. In fact, by some estimates medications are responsible for one in four cases of erectile dysfunction. While there are alternatives that you can explore, remember that your health comes first. Don't discontinue a medication without discussing it with your health care provider first. Great sex becomes meaningless if you die from a heart attack as a result of untreated high blood pressure. If medications are potentially causing sexual dissatisfaction, talk to your doctor about switching to another medication or changing the dose of your existing prescription.

The most common medications that have sexual side effects are some types of antidepressants, high blood pressure medications, antacids, and appetite suppressants. Antidepressants have already been discussed in this chapter. High blood pressure medications, known as antihypertensives, are among the most prescribed medications in the United States. By definition, these medications lower blood pressure, which can also mean that the blood flow to the genitals is reduced. Again, it is important to work directly with your doctor to find acceptable alternatives. See the appendix in the back of this book for a list of common medications known to affect sexual health.

The Bottom Line

Numerous diseases, and the medications used to treat diseases, can put a damper on your sex life.

- Being depressed is the pits for a hearty libido. Likewise, many antidepressants cause a major dip in sexual desire.

- The herb St. John's wort is a natural mood lifter with no sexual side effects.

- Cardiovascular disease can interfere with the proper function of blood vessels feeding the genitals.

- Diabetes is a significant risk factor for erectile dysfunction.

- Other conditions with sexual consequences are

pelvic surgery or trauma, such as hysterectomy, BPH, thyroid conditions, and yeast or bladder infections.

- Getting older often means a greater likelihood of developing a sexual dysfunction.

- Medications are commonly the culprit for libido problems; talk to your doctor about alternative drugs that are kinder to your sex life.

CONCLUSION

By now you've learned that a fulfilling sex life takes more than just popping a Viagra pill. But it also takes more than taking an aphrodisiac herb or dietary supplement. Great sex takes intimacy, communication, good diet choices, a healthy lifestyle, time, and energy. It's common sense, really: If something is good for your overall health, well-being, and relationship, then it is most likely good for your sex life, too.

Sex—like good nutrition, exercise, and mental outlook—contributes to a longer, happier life. In other words, you're never too old for a regular sex life, and in fact, a regular sex life can help you reach old age. In one study of men and women, having sex more frequently led to longer lives in men, while in women *enjoying* sex more led to longer lives. Additional research has confirmed that, for men, death is held at bay when orgasms are more frequent. Modern research confirms that sex is not only fun, it's good for you.

How wonderful that in a world where doctors are constantly telling you what you can't have—cigarettes, eggs, salt, ice cream—there is still something really fun that you have the green light to do as much as you want. So remember, a lot of things go away in older age, but sex shouldn't be one of them. Many older people want and are able to enjoy an active, joyful sex life. Use it or lose it: Regular sexual activity helps maintain sexual ability.

And once the foundation has been set for a healthy sex life—through diet and lifestyle choices—there is no reason not to help guide Cupid's arrows by experimenting with some herbs, vitamins, minerals, and amino acids. As for aphrodisiac foods, whether they work or not is almost beside the point; the mere fact that a couple plans enjoyable time together to experiment with an aphrodisiac may in itself ensure a special night. For no matter which aphrodisiac you try, nothing can match the power of the best aphrodisiac around: the human mind.

COMMON MEDICATIONS WITH SEXUAL SIDE EFFECTS

The following is a list of some of the most commonly prescribed medications that can interfere with sexual function and sexual satisfaction.

Antidepressants

Celexa (citalopram)
Effexor (venlafaxine)
Elavil (amitriptyline)
Luvox (fluvoxamine)
Marplan (isocarboxazid)
Nardil (phenelzine)
Paxil (paroxetine)
Prozac (fluoxetine)
Tofranil (imipramine)
Zoloft (sertraline)
Note: men who suffer from premature ejaculation might benefit from the ejaculation delay caused by antidepressants in the SSRI family.

Antihypertensives

Aldactone (spironolactone)
Aldomet (methyldopa)
Calan (verapamil)
Catapres (clonidine)
Hydropres (reserpine)
Hygroton (chlorthalidone)
Hydrodiuril (hydrochlorothiazide)
Inderal (propranolol)
Ismelin (guanethidine)
Lopressor (metoprolol)

Asthma

Primatene Mist
Atrovent (ipratropium bromide)

Antianxiety

Xanax (alprazolam)
Valium (diazepam)
Ativan (lorazepam)
Librium (chlordiazepoxide)
Restoril (temazepam)

Antiulcer

Axid (nizatidine)
Pepcid (famotidine)
Tagamet (cimetidine)
Zantac (ranitidine)

Birth Control Pills

Ortho-Novum 1/35
Norinyl 1+35
Brevicon
Modicon
Ovcon 35

Cardiac Conditions

Atromid-S (clofibrate)
Lopid (gemfibrozil)
Lanoxin (digoxin)
Apresoline (hydralazine)

Cold/Allergy

Chlor-Trimeton
Benadryl
Excedrin PM
Sudafed

Hormones

Casodex (bicalutamide)
Corticosteroids
Estrogens
Eulexin (flutamide)
Lupron (leuprolide)
Progesterone
Proscar (finasteride)
Zoladex (goserelin)

Miscellaneous

Dexedrine (dextro-
    amphetamine)
Haldol (haloperidol)
Nonsteroidal anti-
    inflammatory drugs
Phenothiazines

SELECTED REFERENCES

Adimoelja A. Phytochemicals and the breakthrough of traditional herbs in the management of sexual dysfunctions. *Int J Androl,* 2000; 23 Suppl 2:82–84.

Bayer R. Treatment of infertility with vitamin E. *Internat J Fertil,* 1960; 5:70–78.

Carey MP, Johnson BT. Effectiveness of yohimbine in the treatment of erectile disorder: Four meta-analytic integrations. *Arch Sex Behav,* 1996; 25(4): 341–60.

Choi HK. Safety and efficacy study with various doses of SS cream in patients with premature ejaculation. *Int J Impot Res,* 1995; 11:261–64.

Choi HK, Seong DH, Rha KH. Clinical efficacy of Korean red ginseng for erectile dysfunction. *Int J Impot Res,* 1995; 7(3):181–86.

Cicero AF, Bandieri E, Arletti R. Lepidium meyenii Walp. Improves sexual behaviour in male rats independently from its action on spontaneous locomotor activity. *J Ethnopharmacol,* 2001; 75:225–29.

Cohen AJ, Bartlik B. Ginkgo biloba for antidepressant-induced sexual dysfunction. *J Sex Marital Ther,* 1998; 24:139–43.

Czeizel AE, Metneki J, Dudas I. The effect of preconceptional multivitamin supplementation on fertility. *Internat J Vit Nutr Res,* 1995; 66:55–58.

Dawson EB, Harris WA, Powell LC. Relationship between ascorbic acid and male fertility. *World Rev Nutr Diet,* 1990; 62:1–26.

Ernst E, Pittler MH. Yohimbine for erectile dysfunction: a systematic review and meta-analysis of randomized clinical trials. *J Urol,* 1998; 159:433–36.

Gillis CN. Panax ginseng pharmacology: A nitric oxide link? *Biochem Pharmacol,* 1997; 54(1):1–8.

Gonzales GF, Cordova A, Gonzales C, et al. Lepidium meyenii (maca) improved semen parameters in adult men. *Asian J Androl,* 2001; 3:301–3.

Guay AT, Jacobson J. Decreased free testosterone and dehydroepiandrosterone-sulfate (DHEA-S) levels in women with decreased libido. *J Sex Marital Ther,* 2002; 28:129–42S.

Hunt C, Johnson P, Herbel J, et al. Effects of dietary zinc depletion on seminal volume and zinc loss, serum testosterone concentrations, and sperm morphology in young men. *Am J Clin Nutr,* 1992; 56: 148–57.

Ito TY, Trant AS, Polan ML. A double-blind placebo-controlled study of ArginMax, a nutritional supplement for enhancement of female sexual function. *J Sex Marital Ther,* 2001; 27:541–49.

Kumar R, Gupta NP. Lycopene therapy in idiopathic male infertility: Results of a clinical trial. Department of Urology, All India Institute of Medical Sciences, New Delhi, 2001.

Lake Polan M. Untitled abstract. *J Women's Health Gender-Based Med,* 2001; 10:401.

Pittler MH, Ernst E. Efficacy of kava extract for treating anxiety: systematic review and meta-analysis. *J Clin Psychopharmacol,* 2000; 20:84–89.

Rowland DL, Kallan K, Slob AK. Yohimbine, erectile capacity, and sexual response in men. *Arch Sex Behav,* 1997; 26:49–62.

Rushton DH, Ramsay ID, Gilkes JJ, et al. Ferritin and fertility. *Lancet,* 1991; 337:1554.

Sandler B, Faragher B. Treatment of oligospermia with vitamin B_{12}. *Infertility*, 1984; 7:133–38.

Sieve BF. The clinical effects of a new B complex factor, para-aminobenzoic acid, on pigmentation and fertility. *South Med Surg*, 1942; 104:135–39.

Sikora R, Sohn M, Deutz FJ, et al. Ginkgo biloba extract in the therapy of erectile dysfunction. *J Urology*, 1989; 141:188A.

Stephens FO. The rising incidence of breast cancer in women and prostate cancer in men. Dietary influences: a possible preventive role for nature's sex hormone modifiers—the phytoestrogens. *Oncol Rep*, 1999; 6:865–70.

Vitali G, Parente R, Melotti C. Carnitine supplementation in human idiopathic asthenospermia: clinical results. *Drugs Exp Clin Res*, 1995; 21:157–59.

Waynberg J, Brewer S. Effects of Herbal vX on libido and sexual activity in premenopausal and post-menopausal women. *Adv Ther*, 2000; 17:255–62.

Zorgniotti AW, Lizza EF. Effect of large doses of the nitric oxide precursor, L-arginine, on erectile dysfunction. *Int J Impot Res*, 1994; 6:33–35.

OTHER BOOKS AND RESOURCES

Reichman, Judith. *I'm Not in the Mood.* New York: William Morrow and Company, 1998.

Wuh, Hank CK and Fox, MeiMei. *Sexual Fitness.* New York: Putnam, 2001.

GreatLife Magazine
Consumer magazine with articles on vitamins, minerals, herbs, and foods.
Available for free at many health and natural food stores.

Let's Live Magazine
Consumer magazine with emphasis on the health benefits of vitamins, minerals, and herbs.
Customer service:
1-800-676-4333
P.O. Box 74908
Los Angeles, CA 90004
Subscriptions: 12 issues per year, $19.95 in the U.S.; $31.95 outside the U.S.

Physical Magazine
Magazine oriented to body builders and other serious athletes.
Customer service:
1-800-676-4333
P.O. Box 74908
Los Angeles, CA 90004
Subscriptions: 12 issues per year, $19.95 in the U.S.; $31.95 outside the U.S.

The Nutrition Reporter™ newsletter
Monthly newsletter that summarizes recent medical research on vitamins, minerals, and herbs.

Customer service:
P.O. Box 30246
Tucson, AZ 85751-0246
e-mail: jack@thenutritionreporter.com
www.nutritionreporter.com

Subscriptions: $26 per year (12 issues) in the U.S.; $32 U.S. or $48 CNC for Canada; $38 for other countries.

Websites

American Association of Sex Educators, Counselors, and Therapists
www.aasect.org
Resource to find a counselor in your area.

The International Council on Infertility Information Dissemination, Inc.
www.inciid.org
Resource for infertility information.

INDEX

Accidents as cause of ED, 52, 69–70
Adaptogens, 14, 17
Adrenal glands, 28
Aging, 53, 73–76
Alcohol, 5–6
  as sex enhancement, 5
  as sex depressant, 5
Almonds, 8
Amazon, 19
Anatomy basics, 33–34
Andropause, 73–74
Antidepressants, 67–68, 77
Antihypertensives, 77
Aphrodisiacs, 4–11, 12–22
  avoiding dangerous, 21–22
  natural, 12–22
Aphrodite, 7, 9, 12
Arabs, 10
Arginine, 8, 12–13, 55, 66
Arousal, 34
  disorder, 38, 40
Art of Love, 8
Artichokes, 10
Asparagus, 10
Atherosclerosis, 68
Attachment phase, 44
Ayurveda, 19, 20
Aztecs, 6

Bananas, 7
Basal temperature, 62
Beans, 6
Bear sex organs, 9
Beetles, 21, 22

Benign prostatic hyperplasia. *See* BPH.
Bicycle riding caution, 25–26
Black cohosh, 76
Blood flow, 15
Blood pressure, high, 32, 69, 77
BPH, 70–71
Breasts, 34
Brevicon, 74

Cardiovascular disease, 40, 52, 57, 58, 69
Cardiovascular fitness, 24
Carnitine, 66
Casanova, 6, 9
Celery, 10
Ceres, 8
Cernilton, 71–72
Cervix, 63–64
Chaste tree berries. *See* Vitex.
Cherries, 7
Chilies, 7
Chinese angelica. *See* Dong quai.
Chinese ginseng. *See* Ginseng, Asian.
Chinese Materia Medica, 15
Chocolate, 6
Cholesterol, high, 23, 32
Cholinergic neurotransmitters, 17
Cialis, 55
Cinnamon, 7
Clitoris, 33, 34, 41, 42

stimulation, 34, 41
Coenzyme Q$_{10}$, 65
Curries, 7

Damiana, 13–14
Dehydroepiandrosterone.
    See DHEA.
Depression, 67–68
Desire, 34
    low, 40
DHEA, 14, 38
Diabetes, 52, 58, 69
Dionysus, 8
Doctors, 55–59, 62–64,
    67–68
    and ED, 55–59
    and infertility, 62–64
    and sex, 67–68
Dole, Bob, 58
Dong quai, 14–15
Dyspareunia, 37, 41

ED, 12, 16, 21, 26, 30, 38,
    39, 51–60, 68, 69–72,
    73–74
    aging and, 53, 73–74
    causes of, 51–53
    doctor
    recommendations,
    55–59
    herbal remedies for,
    53–55
    physical causes of,
    52–53
    primary, 51
    psychological causes
    of, 52–53
    secondary, 51
    smoking and, 30
Eggplants, 11
Egyptians, 8, 10
Ejaculation, 35, 39
Endangered species, 9
Endometriosis, 63
Endorphins, 24
Epimedium. *See* Horny
    goat weed.
Erectile dysfunction.
    See ED.

Eros, 9
EROS–CTD, 42
Eleuthero. *See* Ginseng,
    Siberian.
Emotional attachment
    stage, 44
Erogenous zones, 47, 49
Estrogen, 36, 75
    replacement therapy,
    76
Exercise, 24–27, 32
    routines, 25
    See also Bicycle riding
    caution; Kegels;
    Weight management.

Fallopian tubes, 34, 63
Fantasies, 49
Fat, 23
Fatigue, 30–31
FDA. *See* Food and Drug
    Administration.
Fennel, 8
Figs, 7
Flush, sex, 34
Food and Drug
    Administration, 42, 55
Foods, 4–11, 23–24, 48
    sexually shaped, 4, 10
Fruit, 6, 24

Garlic, 8
Ginger, 7
Ginkgo, 15–16, 54
Ginseng, 16–17, 54
    American, 17
    Asian, 17
    "female," 14
    Siberian, 17
Glans, 33
Gluten, 19–20
Grains, 24
Greeks, 7, 8, 10, 12

Heart attacks, 69
Heart rate, 34
Herbs, 7–8
Hindus, 8, 10

Hormone replacement therapy, 36–38, 75–76
  caution against, 37
Hormones, 36–38
Horny goat weed, 17–18
Hot flashes, 75
HRT. *See* Hormone replacement therapy.
Hysterectomy, 72
Hysterosalpingogram, 63

India, 18
Infatuation stage, 44
Infertility, 61–66
  female, 63–64
  male, 63, 65
Insomnia, 30–31
Institute for Advanced Study of Human Sexuality, 19
Intimacy, 43–50
  creating, 43–50
  stages of, 44
  touch and, 45–47
  trouble with, 44–45
Intracavemous injection, 55–56

Kama Sutra, 10
Kava, 18, 28–29, 55
Kegel, Arnold, 26
Kegels (exercise), 26–27
Korean ginseng. *See* Ginseng, Asian.

Labia, 33, 34, 40
Libido, low, 38, 39
Licorice, 22
Lifestyle, 23–32
Long-term relationships, 44
Luteal phase, 64
Lycopene, 10, 66

Maca, 18
Mace, 7
Magnesium, 29
Mangoes, 7
MAO inhibitors, 16, 17

Massachusetts Male Aging Study, 53
Massage, 46–47
  techniques, 46–47
Masturbation, 36
Mead, 5
Medications, 52, 55–59, 76, 81–82
  as cause of ED, 52
  as cause of sexual dysfunction, 76
Meditation, 27
Menopause, 15, 37, 75–76
Men's sex concerns, 39, 43–50, 73–74
Menstrual cycle, 37, 61–64, 74
  charting, 61–62
Middles Ages, 5, 7, 8, 10
Mineral supplements, 64
Mint, 8
Modicon, 74
Mons Pubis, 33
Montezuma, 6
Mucuna pruriens, 18–19
Muira puama, 19, 55
Music, 48

Nervous system damage, 72–73
Nettles, Stinging, 71
Neurotransmitters, 29
New York University, 12
Nipples, 34, 40
Nitrate drugs, 59
Nitric oxide, 12
Nutmeg, 7
Nutrition, 23–24
Nuts, 8, 24

Oats, 19
Onions, 10
Organs, sex, 9
Orgasms, 34, 35
  difficulties, 35, 38, 40
  multiple, 35
  women and, 35, 40
Ottoman Empire, 16

Ovaries, 34
Ovcon, 74
Ovid, 8
Ovulation, 62–63
Oxytocin, 45
Oysters, 9

PABA, 65
Pacific Islanders, 18, 28
Pain during intercourse, 38, 41
Panax. See Ginseng, Asian.
Pap smear, 63
PDE5, 57
Peaches, 7
Pelvic surgery, female, 72
Penile prosthesis, 56
Penis, 33–35, 39
Peripheral nervous system, 69
Peru, 18
Peyronie's disease, 72
Pfizer, 57
PGE1, 55
Phenylethylamine, 6
Pheromones, 38, 47
Pine nuts, 8
Pistachios, 8
Placebo, 13
PMS, 15, 37
Pollen extract, 71–72
Pomegranates, 7
Potatoes, 10
Pregnancy, 61–66, 74
Premature ejaculation, 15, 38, 39
Premenstrual syndrome. See PMS.
Progesterone, 36–37, 64
Proscar, 70
Prostaglandin E1. See PGE1.
Prostate gland, 70–72
Protodioscin, 20
Pubococcygeal muscles, 26–27
Pygeum, 71

Quince, 7

Reconnecting with partner, 43–50
Refractory phase, 73
Relationships, 43–50
    long-term, 44
    stages of, 44
    troubles with, 44–45
Reproduction, 61–66
Resolution, 34, 35
Rhinoceros horn, 9
Romans, 7, 8, 9, 10

St. Jerome, 6
St. John's wort, 68
Saw palmetto, 71
Scents, 47
Scrotum, 33
Seeds, 24
Self assertion, 48–49
Self understanding, 47
Semen, 33
Sex, 1–3, 4–11, 12–22, 23–32, 33–42, 43–50, 51–60, 61–66, 67–78, 79–80
    aphrodisiacs and, 12–22
    arousal, 34
    doctors and, 67–78
    ED and, 51–60
    exercise and, 24–27
    fatigue and, 30–31
    flush, 34
    foods and, 4–11, 23–24
    hormones and, 36–38
    infertility and, 61–66
    intimacy and, 43–50
    lifestyle and, 23–32
    men's concerns, 39
    primer on, 33–42
    reproduction and, 61–66
    response cycle, 34
    "right amount," 35–36
    sleep and, 30–31
    smoking and, 30
    stress and, 27–30
    techniques, 49–50
    touch and, 45–47

weight management and, 31–32

"what goes wrong," 38

women's concerns, 39–42

Sexual dysfunction, 38, 39–42, 43, 51–60, 67–77

embarrassment over, 43

medical causes, 67–78

Shakespeare, William, 5, 8

Sildenafil. *See* Viagra.

Sleep, 30–31, 53

REM, 53

Smoking, 30, 40

Spanish fly, 21

Sperm, 33

agglutination, 65

count, 63, 65

Spices, 7–8

Squeeze technique, 39

Standardized herbal extracts, 16

Strawberries, 7

Stress, 18, 27–30

management, 27–28

supplements, 28–30

Sunflower seeds, 8

Surgery, 52, 56, 69–70, 72

as cause of ED, 52, 69–70

female pelvic, 72

Testicles, 33, 34

Testosterone, 4, 14, 17, 37–38, 73

Thyroid conditions, 72

Tiger sex organs, 9

Toad venom, 22

Tomatoes, 10

Touch, 45–47, 49

Tribulus, 20, 55

Truffles, 9

Tyramine, 21

Urethral suppositories, 56

Urinary tract infections, 73

Uterus, 34

Vacuum pumps, 56

Vagina, 34, 40

Vaginal lubrication, 34, 40, 74, 75

Vaginal mucus, 62

Vaginismus, 41

Valentine's Day, 6

Valium, 30

Vardenafil, 55

Vegetables, 10, 24

Velvet bean. *See* Mucuna pruriens.

Venus, 7

Viagra, 43, 55–59

colorblindness and, 59

nitrate drugs and, 59

side effects, 58–59

women and, 59

Visual stimuli, 48

Visualization, 28

Vitamins, 64–66

vitamin B complex, 29–30, 64

vitamin B_{12}, 65

vitamin C, 65

vitamin E, 65

Vitex, 20

Vulva, 33

Walnuts, 8

Weight management, 31–32

Wellbutrin, 68

West Africa, 20

Women's sex concerns, 30–42, 43–50, 59, 61–64, 74–75

Yeast infections, 73

Yin yang huo. *See* Horny goat weed.

Yohimbe, 20, 54

Yohimbine, 20, 54

Zinc, 9, 65